MW00694598

"Ron Sandison is cut from the ˍˍˍˍ ˍˍ ˍˍˍˍ ˍˍˍ ˍˍˍˍ ˍˍˍˍˍˍˍˍ ˍˍˍˍ celebrate the strengths of living boldly on the spectrum. These inspirational and loving stories should encourage all who are living, or loving someone, on the spectrum. Thank you for this resource!"

Frank W. Gaskill, PhD, host of the *Dr. G. Aspie Show*

"Everyone should read Ron's book for his heart. We have to listen to adults who showcase neurodiversity. Ron does it beautifully."

Kristine Barnett, best-selling author of *The Spark: A Mother's Story of Nurturing, Genius, and Autism*

"In this unique compilation of compelling reflections, Ron Sandison offers readers new narratives about autism and parenting. These diverse stories are an invitation to listen, ponder, pray, praise, and journey forward in faith."

Erik Carter, PhD, Cornelius Vanderbilt Professor of Special Education at Vanderbilt University

"Everyone is uniquely different, whether a family member, friend, or you yourself have a diagnosis of autism. *Views from the Spectrum* lets you into the world of many autistic individuals, their family life, and how they navigate their day-to-day lives. Every chapter gives a true, positive account and enlightens you on how each individual handles their autism and how wonderful they all really are. This book offers hope and encouragement and gives useful tips and strategies for practical parenting."

Anna Kennedy, OBE, autism ambassador

"*Views from the Spectrum* weaves stories from Ron Sandison's life, and from others with autism spectrum disorders, with biblical truths, practical advice, and spiritual guidance. He writes with great insight, honesty, and humor, combining narrative storytelling skills and theological wisdom. Families blessed with a child with autism: this is your book."

Katherine G. Hobbs, teacher, and writer and researcher for *Autism Parenting Magazine*

"Ron Sandison serves as a needed tour guide and translator for the inner mind of the autistic: a rare gift for parents of nonverbal children with autism. In a cultural landscape where the few mainstream examples of autistics are Dr. Temple Grandin and *Rain Man*, *Views from the Spectrum* offers a refreshing departure from the standard approach of fixating on the remediation of deficiencies, instead encouraging parents to harness and develop their child's unique interests and God-given gifts. Sandison celebrates achievements as unique as each individual through a hopeful show-and-tell of victory stories. Parents like me have much to learn from Ron, his mother, and the Sandison family on how to partner with God and our children to maximize their potential."

Diane Dokko Kim, disability ministry consultant and author of
Unbroken Faith: Spiritual Recovery for the Special Needs Parent

"Ron Sandison has written another must-read book. In *Views from the Spectrum*, Ron has created a lovely introductory text for parents who are either new to autism or interested in learning more from the experts in the field: individuals on the spectrum. As usual, Ron writes about human differences from the inside out and shines a light on autism and all its beauty, gifts, challenges, and wonder. The stories are fantastic, the tone is uplifting, and the insights are beyond valuable. Get this book. Enjoy it, learn from it, and pass it on to someone else needing this powerful perspective."

Paula Kluth, PhD, author of *"You're Going to Love This Kid!"*
and *Pedro's Whale*

"*Views from the Spectrum* reflects the distinctive perspective of Ron Sandison. He describes the time and energy his parents poured into him after he was diagnosed with autism so that he could develop to his full potential. Lest readers think his story is one of a kind, Sandison highlights the accomplishments of other individuals with autism in every chapter. He also weaves practical parenting advice and biblical wisdom throughout the book. This will be an encouraging resource for the autism community and an enlightening one for those who want to support them."

Jolene Philo, coauthor of *Sharing Love Abundantly in Special Needs Families*, national speaker, and host of DifferentDream.com

"Ron's book on autism is invaluable for the Christian parent, teacher, caregiver, or church leader. I love his practical explanations of the multifaceted components of autism, the personal stories he includes, and the biblical principles for parenting, educating, and loving a child with autism. This will be a resource on my shelf as a therapist and would have also been on my school counselor and teacher shelves when I worked in those roles!"

Brenda L. Yoder, LMHC, counselor, educator, licensed school counselor, and parent

"You don't have to be a person of faith to absorb Sandison's faith-based lessons for parents and individuals on the spectrum. In addition to chronicling his own life, he recounts deeply moving stories about how God, love, and perseverance have shaped the lives of people on the spectrum and their families."

Judith Newman, best-selling author of *To Siri with Love: A Mother, Her Autistic Son, and the Kindness of Machines*

"Ron Sandison offers an expert's perspective for parents of autistic children because of his personal experience of growing up with autism. Like few others, he sharply articulates the combustion of passion, family, and faith that spurs an individual with autism on to a purpose-filled life—while at the same time helping caregivers navigate autism's paradoxes. The stories of artists, athletes, and creators that Ron gathers in this book lift up the creative forces of hope and the remarkable, God-given gifts that help the autistic person to emerge and thrive. As a mother of a teenage son with autism, I am encouraged to not grow weary in my efforts to access his rich inner world, helping help him to express it outwardly for a humanity that needs to hear his voice and the voices of other autistic individuals."

Tahni Cullen, best-selling author of *Josiah's Fire: Autism Stole His Words, God Gave Him a Voice*

Views from the Spectrum

Julia, God's
blessings and
favor,
1 Corinthians
13:13

Ron

Sanders

5-22-22

Views from the Spectrum

A Window into Life and Faith with Your Neurodivergent Child

RON SANDISON

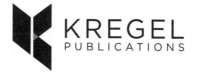

KREGEL
PUBLICATIONS

Views from the Spectrum: A Window into Life and Faith with Your Neurodivergent Child
© 2021 by Ron Sandison

Published by Kregel Publications, a division of Kregel Inc., 2450 Oak Industrial Dr. NE, Grand Rapids, MI 49505.

All rights reserved. No part of this book may be reproduced, stored in a retrieval system, or transmitted in any form or by any means—electronic, mechanical, photocopy, recording, or otherwise—without written permission of the publisher, except for brief quotations in reviews.

Distribution of digital editions of this book in any format via the internet or any other means without the publisher's written permission or by license agreement is a violation of copyright law and is subject to substantial fines and penalties. Thank you for supporting the author's rights by purchasing only authorized editions.

All stories have been supplied by Ron Sandison, and permission for use of these materials is the responsibility of the author. Some names and details have been changed to protect individuals' privacy.

This book is not intended to provide therapy, counseling, clinical advice, or treatment or to take the place of clinical advice or treatment from your personal physician or professional medical health provider. Readers are advised to consult their own qualified health-care physician regarding mental health or medical issues. Neither the publisher nor the author takes any responsibility for any possible consequences from any treatment, action, or application of information in this book to the reader. When a doctor's advice to a particular individual conflicts with the experiences and ideas presented in this book, that individual should always follow the doctor's advice.

All Scripture quotations, unless otherwise indicated, are from the Holy Bible, New International Version®, NIV®. Copyright © 1973, 1978, 1984, 2011 by Biblica, Inc.™ Used by permission of Zondervan. All rights reserved worldwide. www.zondervan.com. The "NIV" and "New International Version" are trademarks registered in the United States Patent and Trademark Office by Biblica, Inc.™

Scripture quotations marked KJV are from the King James Version.

Scripture quotations marked NKJV are from the New King James Version®. Copyright © 1982 by Thomas Nelson. Used by permission. All rights reserved.

Scripture quotations marked NLT are from the Holy Bible, New Living Translation, copyright © 1996, 2004, 2015 by Tyndale House Foundation. Used by permission of Tyndale House Publishers, Inc., Carol Stream, Illinois 60188. All rights reserved.

Cataloging-in-Publication Data is on file with the Library of Congress.

ISBN 978-0-8254-4667-2, print
ISBN 978-0-8254-7717-1, epub

Printed in the United States of America
21 22 23 24 25 26 27 28 29 30 / 5 4 3 2 1

In loving memory of my father-in-law, Bob Boswell (1944–2018). Bob's faith and love in Christ and for his family were evident by his life and actions. He was the perfect father-in-law.

But generous people plan to do what is generous, and they stand firm in their generosity.
—Isaiah 32:8 (NLT)

My beautiful wife, Kristen Sandison, and our daughter, Makayla. For believing in my dreams and providing me time to write and speak.

You should clothe yourselves instead with the beauty that comes from within, the unfading beauty of a gentle and quiet spirit, which is so precious to God.
—1 Peter 3:4 (NLT)

My parents, Chuck and Janet Sandison, for teaching me to pray and trust God. During my dark times of autism and depression, my parents always helped me to overcome and grow in my faith in Christ.

Train up a child in the way he should go: and when he is old, he will not depart from it.
—Proverbs 22:6 (KJV)

My mother-in-law, Sue Boswell, for your love and support.

A generous person will prosper; whoever refreshes others will be refreshed.
—Proverbs 11:25

Contents

Part 4: Resting in God

Foreword

THIS IS A valuable book written by a very qualified author. It is not *about* autism; it is a book that *is* autism personified as told by Ron Sandison through his emergence from his own late-onset autism, and as experienced through the life journeys of twenty other individuals on the spectrum. Ron has become a trusted, plain-speaking, practical advocate for better understanding and helping persons on the spectrum develop their full potential. The twenty other individuals on the spectrum have very special skills ranging from art, poetry, music, and billiard trick mastery to video game design, NASCAR driving, tennis, and baseball.

This book convincingly points out that special skills in persons with autism are not frivolous or circus act curiosities. They are instead "islands of intactness" of various sizes and depth which, when engaged properly, especially by parents who discover, nourish, and celebrate them, can lead to improved communication, socialization, and daily living skills, eventually ending in greater independence.

My introduction to autism was sixty years ago when I had the privilege of learning about it from Dr. Leo Kanner, who first described the condition in 1943. He was a grandfatherly pediatrician who had deep respect for and insights into his patients. He lectured periodically when visiting the medical school in Madison, Wisconsin, where I was a student. I gained from him a great deal of information as well as a gentle bedside manner. It kindled my interest in autism.

My first introduction to an autistic child, however, was not quite as gentle. It was a young girl in a helmet who was banging her head on a table so hard that the rafters shook in the house where the child psychiatry department was located. Yet as I looked at her turmoil and disability, it occurred to me that somewhere, however deeply buried and hidden, there must be some islands of intactness which could be identified, approached, and used to turn adversity into opportunity for learning and healing.

I then went on to start a children's unit at a psychiatric hospital in Wisconsin. It was there that we made a concerted effort to find that island of intactness in each child. We would coax that island closer to the surface, love it, expand it, reinforce it, reward it, and celebrate it. Slowly, better language, improved socialization, increased daily living skills, and eventually greater independence would emerge.

In *Views from the Spectrum* that same basic formula is applied. Parents, grandparents, siblings, or other caregivers search for that island of intactness, whatever size and shape. Whenever discovered, they tend and grow that intactness—that is, the gifts or abilities the individual with autism has despite his or her disabilities—to its fullest extent. That search begins with love—unconditional love—and as I advise the many parents who tell me proudly about their child, "Love is a good therapist too."

There are additional elements in that helping equation that this book describes in detail: patience, untiring perseverance, advocacy, belief, optimism, faith, and hope. In a sense, *Views from the Spectrum* is really two books. The first is Ron Sandison's journey from being able at one point to say only one word, "Mum"—after losing his prior normal developmental milestones—and his inspiring trek back, guided by a loving and intuitive mom using art and a toy prairie dog to help him deal with sensory issues, develop speech, and interact socially.

The other book within this book is about the unique journeys of other persons with autism toward their more optimal fulfillment. In both cases this book, unlike so many others, provides many examples of specific "what to do and how to do it" hints, tips, and pearls for families, therapists, or other caregivers to help them reach the buried potential in each of those persons they love. Refreshingly, the book is free of confusing "psych speak" and lofty theories. Instead it uses everyday language and provides practical ideas as a sort of user manual for parents or families so often overwhelmed and bewildered by the exceptional ability and disability they see in the same person. It advises, correctly, to concentrate on strengths rather than deficits, and to celebrate what is there rather than regret what is missing.

The numerous examples in this book underscore the fact that so often parents, using love, intuition, and creativity, come up with ways to connect with and help their child. That echoes my experience that, in many ways, parents are the real experts on their child. Therefore, professionals need to listen to Mom and Dad more closely to truly grasp the uniqueness of each individual.

Throughout this book the roles of prayer, belief, and faith are included as important elements in the goal of realizing the full potential in these persons with their curious mix of giftedness and limitation.

Overall the book provides much welcomed help and hope. Today there is increasing focus on recognizing strengths rather than deficits in persons with autism, and this book contributes mightily to the implementation of that welcome awakening. This strategy is being applied to persons wherever they appear on the spectrum, whether children or young adults, with the goal to add happiness to the help and hope that this book generously provides.

DAROLD A. TREFFERT, MD
The Treffert Center
www.agnesian.com/services/treffert-center

Introduction

Parenting a child with autism is traveling life's journey with a
different map. Autism does not come with a manual. Instead, it
requires a caregiver who never gives up.

—RON SANDISON

"Though the mountains be shaken and the hills be removed, yet
my unfailing love for you will not be shaken nor my covenant of
peace be removed," says the LORD, who has compassion on you.

—ISAIAH 54:10

WHEN I WAS a child, every year my dad took our family to the Detroit auto show. As an inquisitive seven-year-old, I secretly hurried off to view the newest models of vehicles. After about ten minutes checking out the Corvettes and not paying attention to my family, I suddenly realized I was lost. As panic took over, I fell to the ground and began to cry.

Seeing my distress, two kind gentlemen approached me and said, "Son, don't worry. We'll help you." They gently took my hands and led me through the aisles in search of my family.

My parents and brothers were already desperately looking for me, and after ten minutes I finally saw my dad and ran into his arms, wiping tears onto his pant leg. My mom then picked me up and held me tightly.

"Your son wandered off and was terrified," the first gentleman said.

"You need to keep an extra watch on this one," the second one told them. My parents thanked them, holding tightly to my hands, too shaken to look at any more vehicles.

Ironically, as we began to exit the auto show, my dad noticed a six-year-old girl alone with her head down, crying. My dad asked her, "Are you lost?" She nodded her head.

"Let's find your mom." He took her hand and led her to the security office, seizing the opportunity to pay the two gentlemen's kindness forward.

As we waited for her parents to arrive, I looked at my dad and said, "Do you think her parents left her here and went home?"

My dad gently lifted my chin and looked me in the eye. "Do you think I would have left you here alone?"

"No," I replied as her parents arrived at the security office, joyfully picking her up in their loving arms. I smiled and gave my dad's hand a squeeze.

This memory always reminds me that if parents who love and care for their children will not abandon them, we can trust God will do the same. God understands our fears and worries and will provide for your child, no matter the circumstances. He will never leave nor forsake your family, so we may boldly say, "The Lord is my helper; I will not be afraid" (Hebrews 13:6).

But not being afraid is easier said than done, especially if you're raising a child with autism. Actress and motivational speaker Holly Robinson Peete, whose son RJ has autism, states, "Almost every parent of a child with autism that I have met shares the same fears and hopes. We pray our teenagers will transition into adulthood with self-reliance, a safe place to live, a job with a compassionate employer. More than anything, we want to be assured that our kids will develop the ability to self-advocate, and that they'll find a trusted community."[1]

These are basic hopes that are not easy to accomplish for everyone. It's important to acknowledge that not every child on the spectrum will progress as much as I have, but there is perspective and ground to be won in every circumstance.

Neurological Wiring

Each of us is wired neurologically different. St. Augustine, a fourth-century theologian, in his classic work *City of God*, bragged about his mentor St. Ambrose, stating, "Ambrose is a genius—he is able to read in his mind without saying words verbally." In the fourth century, only 5 percent of the population were literate, and only 10 percent of those who were literate could read silently. Imagine how different our world would be if we were neurologically wired like people in the fourth century—you're flying in an airplane and everyone is reading his or her text messages out loud. Talk about airing dirty laundry! There'd be no need for *TMZ* gossip.

Sarah Parshall Perry, author of *Sand in My Sandwich*, wrote, "Our family's 'flavor' of autism is not the head-banging kind, but the 'Why is that lady so fat?' in a crowded grocery store kind. It is the breathing in someone's face while they speak because he has no concept of personal space kind. The kind we have is a challenge in its own right, different from those of other children on the spectrum because my children look so normal."[2]

> It's often hard to remember that just because a disability isn't readily evident doesn't mean it doesn't exist.

When I experienced meltdowns as a child, I screamed and banged my head relentlessly against a cement wall, or went completely berserk, destroying everything in my path of terror. Most children are like bottled water; they get frustrated or angry and maybe a little water splashes out. As for me, I am neurologically wired like a Mountain Dew that's just been vigorously shaken—watch out!

As a young child, I also struggled with regulating my sense of fear and anxiety. When I was six years old, I feared our house would catch on fire after seeing the 1974 movie *The Towering Inferno*—I didn't sleep in my own bed for four years after this horrifying event.

Invisible Disability

Because autism is sometimes an invisible disability, it's not uncommon to have someone tell you, "Huh. Your child doesn't look autistic to me." The proper response is, "I am glad he does not appear autistic to you. Would you like to have him over for a visit when he is experiencing a full-blown meltdown or anxiety attack?"

Well, maybe not the "proper" response, but it's surely the honest one. Parenting is tough sometimes! And it's often hard to remember that just because a disability isn't readily evident doesn't mean it doesn't exist.

There's a story I like to think about when people struggle with being empathetic toward those of us on the spectrum.

Two wrinkly men in their late eighties are sitting next to each other on a bench. The first one gripes, "I feel so old. My knees throb from arthritis. I have constant back and neck pain. I can barely move, even with my walker, and I have the eyesight of a bat."

The second one winks and replies, "I feel like a newborn baby."

"What do you mean, Fred? You're nearing ninety! You're no spring chicken."

"I am bald, I have no teeth, and my diaper feels like it is leaking," Fred replies.

While this anecdote is meant to make you laugh, it is also meant to remind us that if we live long enough, we are guaranteed to experience some form of disability, whether it be physical or neurological.

Daniel R. Thomson, a physical therapist, shares, "A label that everyone without a disability wears, whether knowingly or not, is *temporarily able-bodied*. It describes people who are not disabled but live one accident, disease, or event away from disability. The truth is that we are closer to the possibility of disability then we may realize."[3]

As you're assisting your child on the spectrum, it might be helpful to ask yourself how you would like to be helped in a similar situation. Figuring out how to care for a child with autism is by no means an easy task, but knowing we might face some form of helplessness in the future can lend a bit of perspective.

Deborah Reber, author of *Differently Wired*, whose teenage son Asher has Asperger's, shares the struggles of raising an atypical child: "Because there is no playbook and there are very few mentors to show us and our kids how it's done and what moving down this road with confidence, grace, and optimism looks like, fears of future unknowns will continue to be a tremendous source of stress raising atypical kids."[4]

Sometimes the job of parenting a neurodivergent child seems overwhelming, but there are things we can do. We can trust God, continue persevering, and forgive ourselves when we let our bottles get a little shaken up.

Blessings and Brokenness

As parents see their dreams for their child quickly slipping away, discouragement and hopelessness seep into their souls. It's hard enough to deal with the death of a dream without the sleepless nights, behavioral issues, doctor appointments, uneducated schools and neighbors, and myriad other struggles a parent deals with on a daily basis.

Having a child with severe autism may even cause you to question your theology of God's love. After her son Tim was born with Down syndrome, minister Stephanie Hubach reprocessed her theological beliefs and came to this conclusion: "On every level of every dimension of the human experience there is a mixture of both the blessedness of creation and the brokenness of the fall. Disability is essentially a more noticeable form of the brokenness that is common to the human experience—a normal part of life in an abnormal world. It is just a difference of degree along a spectrum that contains difficulty all along its length."[5]

Disabilities can affect a child profoundly; autism is no exception. Imagine being unable to communicate with simple sentences or becoming so overwhelmed, all you can do is kick and scream because you have no control over your body. For many children with autism, intense applied behavior analysis (ABA) therapy is required to teach basic life skills, such as tying shoes or not biting.

Mikey Brannigan won the gold medal for running the metric mile in the 2017 Paralympic Games in Rio, but as a child, he required six months of ABA therapy to learn how to walk beside his mother, Edie, instead of always running ahead of her. Edie describes her family's experience as being trapped in "Autism world."[6]

NBC Nightly News reporter Kate Snow asked Mikey, "Does autism make you a better runner?"

Mikey responded, "A better person!"[7]

Just because a child on the spectrum grows into an adult doesn't mean that meltdowns magically disappear. In fact, I still have occasional "honey badger moments" (more on that later).

Fear and Faith

I know as she was raising me, my mom experienced confusion, fear, and isolation—the dark sides of autism. But her faith in God helped her push past that fear. As Francis of Assisi stated, "All the darkness in the world can't extinguish the light from a single candle."[8] God provides his light and comfort in the darkness of autism and brings us closer to his Son, Jesus.

Diane Dokko Kim, author of Unbroken Faith: Spiritual Recovery for the Special Needs Parent, shares the following about raising her son Jeremy, who has autism: "But had my child been like everyone else, I wouldn't have discovered how passionately I could love, how bitterly I could weep, how desperately I could pray, or how fiercely I could fight. Disabilities demolished my pride and self-sufficiency; it remapped the boundaries of my narrow mind—and even smaller heart—to grow expanses of sorrow, surrender, and submission."[9]

Although our fear for our children and their disabilities is real, we can give thanks that in raising them, we can see disabilities give way to hidden beginnings. Autism has been a paradox for me: both blessing and suffering. As a child, I hated loud noises, yet I was always the loudest child in the room. I graduated from university with a master's degree and perfect 4.0 GPA, but in high school I could not pass Spanish or geography.

I have great attention to detail, recalling childhood memories, yet miss social cues like yawning by disinterested coworkers when I share (what I consider) my humorous psych-ward stories. I speak at more than seventy events a year on autism, yet my supervisor, Dwayne, compares my social filtering system to a child riding a bike barefoot downhill without brakes. Arthur Fleischmann, coauthor of *Carly's Voice: Breaking Through Autism*, describes the autism paradox:

> Everything in our family was lived on extremes. When Carly was home, her presence was enormous and all-consuming. When she was gone [for respite care], I felt empty and hollow. Carly's intelligence far exceeded that of most kids, but her behavior was far below that of the mainstream. The polar extremes were exhausting. One life was too black-and-white, and I yearned for some gray—some in-between.
>
> I hoped that when Carly was away, absence would make the heart grow blinder and in time I would ache less while she was away, and be more at peace when she was home. For the time being we would have to live in a binary world—Carly here or gone—and that would have to be good enough. At least for a little while.[10]

The paradox of living between two extremes can be draining, but try not to worry. Remember that God will provide balance and stability, and you will discover beauty in the autism paradox.

A Story of Two Barns

A pastor was on vacation in the southern United States and noticed a broken and dilapidated red barn next to a field filled with thorns, thistles, and an anorexic cow. He drove another mile up the country road and saw a beautiful red barn with a garden of red roses and a ripe harvest. The pastor approached the farmer and said, "Wow, God has really blessed you with this beautiful farm!"

The farmer looked at the pastor, laughed, and said, "You should have seen the farm when it was only God here!"

Raising a child with special needs requires faith plus hard work and perseverance. St. Augustine wrote, "Pray as if everything depends on God, and work as if everything depends on us."[11]

In other words, you can't just sit around waiting for God to bless you with good fortune. You and God must work as a team.

There were many years when my life appeared more like the rundown barn next to a field of thorns than what you see of me on Facebook or the professional photo on the back of my books that makes me look like an autistic celebrity.

What to Expect

Throughout this book, I'll share many inspiring stories of faith, love, and the courage of young adults with autism and how they, alongside their families, grow closer to God. These young adults shine as mentors offering us hope and guidance to persevere with confidence and grace. With each story, you will learn how to experience God-filled moments and receive his guidance in raising your child.

> Your child is created in the image of God with a purpose and destiny.

The parents I interviewed for this book shared eight characteristics that empowered their children with autism to thrive and overcome learning challenges:

1. Recognize the issues to be tackled.
2. Focus on your child's strengths and abilities.
3. Celebrate your child's progress.
4. Keep a positive attitude.
5. Advocate fiercely for your child.
6. Learn to see the world from your child's perspective.
7. Never give up on your child.
8. Believe that God has a special plan for your child.

As you read, I want to encourage you to pray and trust your child to God. As King Solomon said, "Trust in the LORD with all your heart and lean not on your own understanding; in all your ways submit to him, and he will make your paths straight" (Proverbs 3:5–6).

Remember that God sees the road ahead of you, and he has an amazing plan for your family. Your child is created in the image of God with a purpose and destiny. As you seek God, he will empower you and give you parenting wisdom. Autism humbled my family and enabled us to grow in faith. It made us who we are. God used our struggles to help other families and bring healing. Don't hide your wounds; they're badges of perseverance.

As Romans 15:13 says, "May the God of hope fill you with all joy and peace as you trust in him, so that you may overflow with hope by the power of the Holy Spirit."

God's view on the spectrum is full of hope when you relentlessly pursue him in the darkness, confusion, and fear, trusting him to empower you to raise your child. You will discover God's strength is perfected in your weakness. You'll also discover new friends along the way. I pray this book will provide you with comfort and insight on your journey.

PART 1

Where to Begin

Chapter 1

Real Superheroes Don't Wear Capes

All God's giants have been weak men who did great things for God because they reckoned on God being with them.

—J. HUDSON TAYLOR, MISSIONARY TO CHINA

When you pass through the waters, I will be with you; and when you pass through the rivers, they will not sweep over you. When you walk through the fire, you will not be burned; the flames will not set you ablaze.

—ISAIAH 43:2

SINCE YOU ARE reading this book I'm going to assume that you are a parent or caretaker of a child on the spectrum. You care deeply about that child and part of what drew you to this book is that I, myself, am on the spectrum. Yes, I'm university educated and work in the mental health field, but my best qualification by far is that I live on the spectrum. And my guess is that what you're most interested in are the hard-won successes my parents and I have uncovered.

As a parent of a child with autism and special needs, you understand firsthand the feeling of seeing your child's school office number flash across your phone while you're in an important business meeting. Or you're catching up on email when a message pops up from your child's teacher requesting a conference. Or enjoying coffee with a neighbor when her child runs up screaming because your son pulled out a chunk of her hair. Or listening attentively to your pastor's message on faith and endurance when your daughter's number appears on the monitor, a blatant sign that there is trouble in the nursery.

Curt Warner, a former running back for the Seattle Seahawks and Los Angeles Rams, whose twin sons have autism, writes:

> At times I'd get flashbacks to football games when things were going bad. Sometimes you're getting beaten and there's nothing you can do about it. No matter what you do—the game plan, substitutions, trick plays—you're still just getting a beatdown. What do you do? You have no choice, you've got to line up and try it again. Play after play. The only thing you can do is just keep going back at it and keep trying to do your best. Sometimes you just have days like that. That's pretty much what every day felt like for us for a long time.[1]

My journey with autism has been an amazing adventure of faith and hope, where my parents became my superheroes—conquering the seemingly impossible—and I became their superhero in training.

My development was normal until I reached eighteen months. I began to rapidly regress, losing my ability to communicate with words and ceasing to maintain eye contact. About 20 percent of children with autism experience a period of regression of previously acquired skills as I did, while many others have a developmental delay with communication and fine motor skills.[2]

Because my mom had two neurotypical children before me, she was quick to realize my development and communication abilities were severely delayed and immediately took me to the family pediatrician.

The pediatrician dismissed my mom's concerns, explaining, "Men are like fine wine. You have to give them time to develop. Women are like delicate flowers and blossom quickly."

My mom is not one to wait around. She immediately advocated for me to receive speech therapy. As a result, from ages two to sixteen, I received intense therapy. When I was seven years old, my speech was so delayed, my brother Chuckie bragged to his friends, "You've got to meet my brother Ronnie. I think he is from Norway since he sounds Norwegian!" For a while, Chuckie and the rest of my family were the only ones able to "interpret" my language.

As I entered kindergarten, the Rochester Community Schools specialists wanted to label me as emotionally impaired. My mom refused this label and informed the professionals, "My son's disability is not emotional but neurological." She diligently researched the top professionals for learning disabilities in the area and paid to have me retested. A neuropsychologist from Henry Ford Hospital confirmed that my disability was indeed neurological and defined as autism.

> Love doesn't make everything turn out exactly the way we wish it would every time, but it does make unimaginable growth possible.

When I was diagnosed with autism in 1982, only one in every ten thousand children in the US was so diagnosed. Now one out of fifty-four children is diagnosed, with boys more than four times as often as girls.[3]

The educational specialists and doctors warned my parents that I would never read beyond a seventh-grade level, attend college, excel in athletics, or have meaningful relationships. But my mom was undeterred by these generalities and instead became more determined to help me succeed in life by developing my unique gifts. She helped me gain self-confidence through creative activities such as painting, drawing, reading, and writing short stories.

I now have a bachelor's degree in theology and psychology—earning a 3.9 GPA in the process—and a Master of Divinity with a minor in Koine

Greek from Oral Roberts University. I received an athletic scholarship for track and cross-country my freshman year of college. My wife, Kristen, and I were married on December 7, 2012. On March 20, 2016, my daughter, Makayla Marie, was born, and just a couple of weeks later, Charisma House published my first book, *A Parent's Guide to Autism: Practical Advice. Biblical Wisdom.*

My mother's intuition, persistence, perseverance, commitment, and love accomplished unfathomable things. Of course love doesn't make everything turn out exactly the way we wish it would every time, but it does make unimaginable growth possible.

Both of my parents chose to focus on my abilities and the talents God had given me and, as a result, I flourished. They lived by Dr. Temple Grandin's wisdom: "In special education, there's too much emphasis placed on the deficit and not enough on the strength."[4]

My mom believed that by having me interact with typical children my own age, I would learn essential social skills, and by developing my talents, I could gain independence and accomplish my dreams. She also knew from her research that not every child with autism will gain independence and advocacy for me would be a monumental task, but she knew it was worth the attempt.

Inspired by the wisdom books in the Bible, she often recited to me, "Do you see a man skilled in his work? He will serve before kings; he will not serve before obscure men" (Proverbs 22:29, NIV 1984). With my mom's wisdom and guidance, I homed in on my skills, which has led to a prosperous and fulfilling life.

That quick summary makes it all seem rather easy. But you and I both know it isn't.

My coworker Robert shared a humorous story about his fifteen-year-old cousin, when they were both attending his grandfather's funeral. Cousin Mark, who has Asperger's, is Protestant, has sensory smell issues, and had never been to a Catholic church. As the pallbearers carried his grandfather's casket, the priest conducting the funeral announced, "Please bow your heads and close your eyes for a moment of silence in reverence for the departed." The altar boys followed, waving the thurible as the aroma of incense quickly filled the sanctuary.

In the midst of the silence, Mark screamed, "Who the *hell* would bring incense to a funeral? What the—!" Well, you can imagine the rest. In moments like these you don't think of the word *superhero* to describe your child. In fact, when your son or daughter demonstrates quirky behavior in public, superhero is the last thought on your mind . . . unless you're thinking you are a superhero for containing your reaction. But a superhero can surprise you in the most unlikely moment.

Tyler Gianchetta: A Real-Life Superhero

On July 15, 2015, Susan drove her nineteen-year-old son with high-functioning autism, Tyler, to his doctor appointment in Long Island.[5] As they chatted and enjoyed the summer ride, Susan's body suddenly began to shake uncontrollably, and she became unresponsive. Within moments, their car raced like a derailed train into a tree.

Smoke from the engine instantly began to fill the car as Tyler frantically attempted to break free from the erupting inferno.

"I responded with instinct," Tyler later recalls. "I just kept thinking to myself, 'Don't let Mom die!'"

Breaking loose from his passenger seat, Tyler swiftly smashed the driver's side window with his bare hands and rescued his unconscious mom from the mangled mess.

Thirty seconds after he moved her from the wreckage, the car exploded. Thick black clouds of smoke engulfed the air as the sound of approaching sirens whined in the distance. Tyler lay by the roadside next to his mom who had a shattered hip, broken neck, cracked ribs, and burn injuries.

After being branded a hero in an interview with CBS New York, Tyler declared, "I don't know when my hand got broken. I don't know if it was from the accident or from pulling my mom out. But I can tell you right now that if it was broken pulling her out, I'd break the other hand to pull her out again because I love her so much."[6]

Tyler's surgery required fourteen screws and a small plate in his hand. Susan's doctors were unable to determine the initial cause of her passing out, which had caused the accident.

Reflecting on this moment, Tyler shares, "The hand of God was visible in two ways. First, the car was on a steep incline following the crash, giving me leverage to pull my mom from the vehicle. Second, I was able to open my passenger door. When the insurance company investigated the charred wreckage a few days later, they were unable to open my door. The claim agents were baffled that we were able to escape."

Tyler Gianchetta was developmentally delayed in his communication and fine motor skills and, at two and a half years old, he was diagnosed with high-functioning autism. The Huntington New York public school district wanted him to attend an elementary school with a special education program. "My mom told the district that I would not attend a school twenty minutes away from home, and she insisted that I attend the same school as my friends," Tyler shared. Ironically, years later Tyler served as a teacher's assistant at the very school his mom fought vigilantly for him to attend. From an early age, he persisted in overcoming the odds.

One way that Tyler found to communicate was through music. "Music saved my life," he shares. "As a child, I had trouble expressing myself. I learned self-expression through my passion for music. I learned to talk later than my peers, but I could express myself through music. No matter what I was going through, I could sing about it and feel comfort."

Michael, Tyler's dad, shares with relatives and friends, "Picture a five-year-old child running around the house in his underwear singing and performing Whitesnake's 'Here I Go Again.' That's Tyler!"

Tyler is a fierce advocate for people with disabilities. In high school, he frequently stood up to bullies who were harassing others. He recalls one time when a student was bothering a peer with autism. Tyler had the courage to walk right up and dare the kid to tease him instead because he had autism too. The kid looked completely perplexed and walked away, muttering, "You sure don't look autistic!" You can bet the fellow student with autism saw Tyler as a superhero—he swooped in and protected him from someone stronger and more powerful.

After graduating from high school, Tyler attended Clark University in Worcester, Massachusetts. "I chose to attend Clark because the students are accepting. For example, I wore my New York Islanders jersey to an assembly for orientation and sat next to a fellow student who was wearing his Bruins jersey. After we talked about our passion for hockey, I discovered that he also had autism and before long, I had a new friend."

Tyler graduated with bachelor degrees in mathematics and economics in 2018 from Clark University and is now a successful tax analyst. Tyler still demonstrates his superhero qualities by helping individuals with autism and special needs with their accounting.

Tyler's parents did everything possible to help Tyler thrive in life and education. Reflecting on that miraculous moment after the car crash, Tyler exclaims, "My mom has saved my life dozens of times, and I was finally able to save her life."

True superheroes willingly risk their own lives for others by sacrificing their comfort and safety.

Tyler also advises young people with autism, "Perseverance and knowing your limitations are keys to success. Don't be afraid to ask for help."

Even heroes need a helping hand sometimes.

Five Steps to Developing a Hero

Marvel and DC Comics blockbuster movies portray a superhero as possessing amazing gifts like a robotic outfit to transform a mere man into an ant warrior or a bat cape to glide undetected through Gotham City. However, a real superhero, such as Tyler, is an ordinary person who, in times of crisis, is able to draw forth an extraordinary quality of strength and courage from within to triumph in the midst of severe circumstances. True superheroes willingly risk their own lives for others by sacrificing their comfort and safety. As Jesus taught his disciples, "Greater love has no one than this: to lay down one's life for one's friends" (John 15:13). And every person, no matter their struggles, can sacrifice and have abilities beyond the rest of their peers.

Tyler's story is proof that no matter what our children's struggles are, they have the capacity to be heroes—people who strive to reach their full potential and use their gifts to serve others. What they need is someone strong and heroic in their own right to guide them along. While everyone's journey will look different, I offer five pieces of advice we can all use to help our children become superheroes.

1. Know where super powers come from.
Even Superman is crippled by kryptonite and depends on others to help him. It would be foolish for him to go into battle not knowing his weakness and how to combat it. The same is true for all of us. Real life is full of pitfalls and dangers, but because of their particular struggles, children on the spectrum are especially in danger, and they need us as parents to introduce them to the ultimate power to save them.

A friend of mine, who is a pastor with three children including a son and daughter on the spectrum, encourages his children to stay positive and always trust Jesus. After watching superhero movies, he encourages them, "Jesus is the one mightier than I. He is strong enough to fight your battles. In times of trouble take refuge in him." While building cardboard castles and playing knights in armor, his neurotypical son picked up a plastic sword and said to his brother with Asperger's, "Choose your weapons!"

His brother replied, "I choose Jesus. He is the one mightier than I."

A few weeks later, this pastor took his children to *Avengers: Endgame*. On the ride back from the theater, he asked his children, "What superpower would you want?"

His son with Asperger's exclaimed, "I want Jesus."

"Why?"

"Because Jesus is mightier than I. He already won all the battles. I can take refuge in him."

Don't brush by that statement too quickly. There is powerful truth there. Real-world heroes need God to fully achieve their superhero status. So speak to your children often about God. Make him concrete by telling them the things he has done in your life and theirs. Sing them songs. Read to them from the Bible. Show them how the Bible has changed you and helped you.

2. Model your inner superhero.
Children with autism are great imitators. If you give up, your child with autism will also give up. If you continue to use your gifts to pursue mak-

ing your child the hero they can be, your child will continue to reach for his full potential. The apostle Paul said, "Let us not become weary in doing good, for at the proper time we will reap a harvest if we do not give up" (Galatians 6:9). Second Chronicles 15:7 encourages us, "But as for you, be strong and do not give up, for your work will be rewarded."

My mom refused to lose hope when the special education experts informed her, "Your son will never read beyond a seventh-grade level or attend college." But because she modeled a hero's attitude of never giving up, I chose to be a hero and not give up as well.

Like my mom, Julie Hornok, whose daughter Lizzie has autism, always tries to keep a hope-filled attitude. She says, "I had a choice. I could focus on what my daughter couldn't do or what she could do. Focusing on what she couldn't do had kept me from enjoying her in the moment, and she deserved better than that. She deserved to be loved and adored exactly as she was because she was an incredible little girl. The more I focused on what she could do, the more I was able to use her strengths to support her weaknesses."[7]

Reassessing your child's abilities is important for setting reachable goals. Not every child with autism will gain independence. Some will live in a group home. Your focus is on finding the next potential goal. That could be to have your nonverbal child learn to handle his aggression and not bite, or learn simple sign language to express his immediate needs.

3. Be a force to be reckoned with.

The main characteristic of every superhero is being an advocate for the weak and a person you don't want to confront in combat. When you advocate for your child's IEP or additional resources, he will learn to be an advocate for himself and others too.

Last year the hospital I work at was so understaffed that the CEO and Director of Nursing ordered mandatory overtime for the nursing staff. Being mandated by a supervisor can cause severe anxiety for an employee with autism, as it did for me. In response to the new policy, I self-advocated by having an Oakland University professor of autism write a letter requesting accommodations for my autism under the Americans with Disabilities Act. All my buddies were mandated to work late on

Friday and Saturday nights while I got to go home on time—disabilities sometimes do have benefits.

My mom modeled advocacy by making sure I received every resource from the school system I needed to succeed. Be the parent who is willing to stand up and fight for your child, and keep fighting until your child's voice is heard. Then help another parent stand up. When we all stand together, we are an overwhelming force.

4. Celebrate your child's progress by keeping a journal.

Every superhero needs someone who will share their progress with the world, and it's a rare person who doesn't like being celebrated. You have the opportunity to make your child feel like a superhero by chronicling their successes and struggles that lead to more successes. In a journal or scrapbook, recount how far they have come and the battles they have won, then share these records with your child. Lori Ashley Taylor, author of *Dragonfly: A Daughter's Emergence from Autism*, writes, "I learned to celebrate the smallest successes, because [Hannah] did make progress even when it was minuscule. We celebrated *inchstones* instead of milestones. I believe that's the reason compliments come easy for special needs parents. We notice small accomplishments in big ways."[8]

Celebrating every moment will give you and your child the encouragement to continue to the next small step.

5. Focus on ability and not labels.

Every superhero has strengths and weaknesses. We don't refer to a superhero by their weakness but by their strength. Superman is the Man of Steel, not the man prone to be sick by the kryptonite flu. My mom focused on my abilities, such as art and a powerful memory. She refused to let others' labels hold me back. This taught me to refuse labels and to be a trailblazer in life.

In fact, the labels given in autism—high and low functioning—essentially refer to a person's ability to speak. That's it. It's also true that these labels can, at times, do more harm than good. A low-functioning diagnosis might cause a person to be set aside as unreachable. Yes, a diagnosis can help parents and professionals in knowing what tools might be most effective in helping your child, but they don't tell you anything else about a person on the spectrum and all of their abilities.

Every child has a special ability. As parents, it's up to us to help our children find it and foster it. With the right guidance and support, we all have the potential to be superheroes.

CLOSING THOUGHTS

Our children have unique gifts and disabilities. They are superheroes trying to figure out their abilities and learn to use them to overcome life's challenges. We should not label children but instead be their source of heroic love and support. Love will boost their self-esteem and encourage them to reach new heights.

One more note of encouragement. Like my mom, you also will have moments when you question your child's superpower abilities, and that's okay. You may be your child's hero, but you're also human. The good news is that your source for superhero powers is always available to give you support.

PRAYER AND MEDITATION

Prayer

God, open my eyes to the talents and strengths you've given my child. Bring compassionate teachers and therapists who can refine those gifts and help my child learn social skills and gain independence. Surround us with your favor and love. Teach me patience, for you are my God; I will trust in you. May your good Spirit lead me on level ground and make my steps firm. Amen.

Meditation

> When the servant of the man of God got up and went out early the next morning, an army with horses and chariots had surrounded the city. "Oh no, my lord! What shall we do?" the servant asked.

"Don't be afraid," the prophet answered. "Those who are with us are more than those who are with them."

And Elisha prayed, "Open his eyes, LORD, so that he may see." Then the LORD opened the servant's eyes, and he looked and saw the hills full of horses and chariots of fire all around Elisha. (2 Kings 6:15–17)

Do not forget to entertain strangers, for by so doing some have unwittingly entertained angels. (Hebrews 13:2 NKJV)

Chapter 2

Where Hope Can Be Found

Many things are possible for the person who has hope. Even more
is possible for the person who has faith. And still more is possible
for the person who knows how to love. But everything is possible
for the person who practices all three virtues.

—BROTHER LAWRENCE, SEVENTEENTH-CENTURY FRENCH MONK

Yes, my soul, find rest in God;
my hope comes from him.

—PSALM 62:5

AMERICAN PSYCHOLOGIST DR. Martin Seligman discovered what he
called the hopelessness complex while researching learned helplessness in
1967 at the University of Pennsylvania. Learned helplessness is a behavior that occurs when individuals experience failure enough times that
they believe they are incapable of success, causing them to stop trying.

Dr. Seligman and his partner Dr. Maier were conducting electric
shock experiments on dogs, a highly controversial method by today's
standards. The first group of dogs received a painful shock on the right
side of the lab, learning quickly to move to the left side to avoid the shock

again. The second group received shocks on the left side, so they learned to move to the right. However, the third group was shocked on both sides, so they remained in their spots, intelligent enough to realize that no matter where they moved, they would feel the shock; they learned helplessness.

You and your child with autism may also feel stuck due to a hopelessness complex. At times it will feel like it doesn't matter what you do, and it's painful. Some of the causes for hopelessness include bullying, difficulty with communication from speech deficits, struggles in academics from learning disabilities, a distorted perspective of all-or-nothing thinking, sensory issues, failures in relationships, unemployment, awkward social interactions, and a fear of the future. The roots of the hopelessness complex include despair, lack of motivation, fear of trying new things, depression, anxiety, and other mental health issues.

Faith in God empowered me to have a hope complex and overcome my insecurities.

I understand those feelings. The hopelessness complex dominated my life and thinking for many years, but faith in God empowered me to have a hope complex and overcome my insecurities. Having a hope complex was key for me in developing relationships, finding success in academics, and acquiring gainful employment. As Proverbs 13:12 says, "Hope deferred makes the heart sick, but a longing fulfilled is a tree of life."

Your child too can develop a hope complex! Here are four tips that helped me. Use them as you move your child from hope*less* to hope*ful*!

1. A healthy self-efficacy is key to overcoming hopelessness.

Self-efficacy is a person's *belief* in his or her ability to execute the actions necessary to achieve desired outcomes. Notice that it has little to do with whether or not the person can actually perform an activity right now. Hope is gained when a person believes that he or she can achieve something. And people believe in themselves when other people believe in them. Austin John Jones, a young adult artist with autism, gives this advice on motivation and feeling secure:

> I know that the choices I make shape my life. Sometimes I choose to play video games on my phone when I'm with a group of people because it's easier than trying to talk or listen when a bunch of people are talking. Sometimes I go into my room when my parents have people over because it's better for me to play a video game or talk to just one person online. I do it because I don't have the confidence to sit in a conversation and try to figure it all out. It's easier to not have to worry about it. I know there are consequences when I make a choice like this (at least I am learning that with my parents' help). People might think I'm rude or not interested in them or that I don't love or care about them. But I do.
>
> Making choices can be really scary and it can leave me feeling unsteady and insecure. I want to live life to the fullest. And how can I do that? I have to have confidence in every aspect of my life but that is not easy when you are on the spectrum. I often do things differently than the people around me, and they need to understand that's just who I am. Even though I'm not always good at it, I think it's important to believe in yourself and I am trying all the time to do that.[1]

My self-esteem developed as I interacted socially and learned to express my ideas. Each time my parents encouraged me not to isolate myself in my room when they had guests over helped me achieve small successes. Those small achievements built up until I believed I could interact effectively with others. My parents took the same route of slowly building up my confidence in other areas of my life. Now I have a healthy self-efficacy that allows me to feel confident about most everything in life.

In college, my self-efficacy enabled me to travel on summer mission trips and share the good news of Jesus Christ. I felt confident to visit cool places like Madagascar, Cameroon, France, and Bulgaria and try new foods like eel, spicy toucan, and baboon gumbo. I also was chosen each trip to be the main speaker for our team. Something my early teachers would never have foreseen.

2. A hope complex sees challenges as new opportunities.

When I felt overwhelmed by college papers and assignments, my parents would ask me to share with them why I felt so stressed and what I feared. After praying for God's peace, my dad encouraged me, "Give your best and study, but don't think that you have to get perfect grades. Effort is what counts most, not a professor's grade. What does it matter if you get a C or an A on your paper? Remember, God is in control."

They were teaching me to analyze my all-or-nothing mindset. By encouraging me to verbalize obsessive thought patterns, my parents helped me see new opportunities for solving problems. Things are not just black-and-white (I either get an A or I'm a failure), but also gray (a C is a passing grade and may be the best I can do with what I had on that particular day).

When your child is faced with something that feels overwhelming, help them see it as an opportunity to reach further than they have before. You can do that by teaching your child to break down larger tasks into manageable steps. On a chart or calendar, write down the goal or deadline and work toward it, setting small goals along the way. Don't forget to offer rewards for reaching each goal. Have him or her decide in advance how much time to spend on a task. Remember, the goal is to complete the task, not to make it perfect.

3. The ability to make choices in life creates hope.

Having limited options in making choices leads to a lack of motivation. When you're unemployed, have few friends, no driver's license, and a restricted budget, you become limited in the choices you can make; this can be very depressing for anyone, let alone someone whose struggles are compounded with a disability.

If we can offer choices, though, we can create motivation which will lead to action. Brett, a gentleman in his fifties with autism, refused to leave his room at a group home for days. Staff had bite and scratch marks covering their arms from trying to force him to leave his room. A behavioral therapist visited Brett at lunchtime and told staff, "I think I can get Brett to leave his room." She put two chairs outside his room—a hard chair and a soft chair—and said, "Brett, what chair do you want to sit in?" Brett slowly left his room and *chose* to sit in the soft chair. For years, Brett was given orders, what to do and when to do it, without choice. Given the dignity of choice, Brett was quite willing to move forward.

We also need to remember, especially with children on the spectrum, motivation is not lacking in areas of special interests. If we can incorporate choices that allow for time with their special interests, children with autism can flourish.

4. True hope comes from Christ.

As a child with autism, I often felt hopeless. My daily outlook was, "It's always darkest just before complete and utter darkness." An Eeyore-like depression clouded my every thought. Christ transformed my thinking from a hopelessness complex and gave me hope. As I read the Bible and followed Christ's call on my life, slowly the depression became more bearable. I still experience times of darkness and confusion, but I have learned to seek help from friends and place my hope in Christ.

Colossians 1:27 says, "To them God has chosen to make known among the Gentiles the glorious riches of this mystery, which is Christ in you, the hope of glory." Hope is found in Christ if we follow his call.

Peter Lantz, a young man with Asperger's, took this advice to heart. By following Christ's call, he became a talented video game designer.

Peter Lantz: Using Asperger's for a Career in Video Games

While waiting for my haircut at Great Clips, I struck up a conversation with Peter Lantz, a young adult with Asperger's.[2] Peter works for an advertising company designing video games. As we waited for our haircuts, Peter shared his adventure in following Christ and divine vocation to create educational video games. He is a perfect example of how it's possible for a hope complex to turn a difficult life into a life filled with purpose—following God's call.

"I have a unique job. I work as the only game developer in an advertising agency. I code, create art, and do design work for the games we produce. Sometimes a client wants a virtual reality (VR) experience or something similar, and that's where someone like me comes in. Other times it's research and development or 'showoff' work that helps sell us as an agency. With the advancement of game-creation tools over the years, it's become feasible for one person to throw together very small games as a career.

"When I first read the job description online, it sounded like a job I didn't want. I would be the only game developer at an advertising agency, which meant no one would understand my work and how long it takes. However, when I finally went to the company's website and checked out their values, it became clear this was a strong Christian company that believed 'love was the only rule.' That statement resonated deeply inside, and I instantly suspected God was up to something. I kept seeing phrases related to 'love' everywhere I went and knew for sure God intended me to work at the company."

Peter decided to apply for the job, and with a strong recommendation and portfolio, he landed it. Having a hope complex fueled by a healthy self-efficacy helped him find gainful employment with a job he now loves.

Small Beginnings

Zechariah 4:10 says, "Do not despise these small beginnings" (NLT). In reaching his dream job, Peter had many challenges to overcome. Early in Peter's development, his parents realized by his behavior he had some form of autism and decided to homeschool him. Peter was unable to speak complete sentences until he began working with a speech therapist, then was diagnosed with Asperger's at the age of fourteen.

The DSM-5 defines Asperger's syndrome as a developmental disorder characterized by severely impaired social skills, repetitive behaviors, and often, a narrow set of interests, but not involving delayed development of linguistic and cognitive abilities. Under the DSM-5, Asperger's is part of the autism spectrum disorders.

Asperger's enables Peter to have a great ability to focus, but it comes with a cost. As Peter shared, "If I put my mind to something, it will get done, but the rest of my life always suffers. If I do work on a computer, I hardly get exercise. If I'm getting into a project, I let miscellaneous tasks fall through the cracks like replying to emails or cleaning my apartment."

Asperger's causes Peter to feel misunderstood. "I get the impression people who don't know me well think I have a secret agenda. They feel like I'm hiding something when I talk because I have trouble looking them in the eye. I also feel like I have to choose my words carefully and 'control' what their reaction will be since I am always afraid what I'm saying will be taken wrong, having messed up before in the past. It makes it look like I'm some sort of bad guy. I now know for some people it's just not my fault; they had a chip on their shoulder."

For Peter, the "small beginnings" included social awkwardness, difficulty with communication, feeling misunderstood, and learning disabilities. He was able to overcome these initial struggles with the help of his parents and by using his gifts of focus and perseverance.

After finishing home schooling, Peter attended a local tech center. He enrolled in many technical classes; the ones he enjoyed most were programming, graphic design, and 3D animation.

Peter felt 3D animation was his answer from God to getting a job that suits his natural skills. He met his mentor, Richard Vandermey, at the tech center. Richard encouraged Peter to pursue his dream of designing video games. Taking his advice, he joined a team, placing third in a national competition.

"My parents expressed concern that this industry was only for the extremely skilled, but I kept pushing them since it became a holy war of some kind for me. I knew this was where God wanted me. I knew this was what I wanted to do, so they let me enroll in Ferris State University."

College Success

Peter's parents helped prepare him for college by saving money in a college trust fund. Once enrolled at Ferris, Peter's speech therapist met with him weekly, teaching him how to analyze stories and then share his ideas in essay form. Peter's dad helped him learn to write business letters, preparing him for technical writing.

"I lived at home during college, so I got to eat my mom's delicious home cooking and save on room and board. Mentally, I may not have been ready to be independent yet, so staying at home gave me some time."

Peter's favorite college classes at Ferris State were the 3D art. He loved working with spatial relationships and creating interactive video game art. "I was the star student since the program, Digital Animation and Game Design, fit me like a glove. Within the first semester I achieved every goal I set out to do. I joined the game development club, I earned an award for my classwork, and I attended the Game Developer's Conference as a volunteer (which I ended up doing every year afterward, to this day).

"My first years of college were amazing. I learned how to work hard in front of a computer and had two extremely competent art professors directly from the game industry. One would share his knowledge of game development after class, responding to question after question I sent his way. I learned a ton those years.

"I was often given the freedom to change up assignments if I wanted to try something different in a class since I was a good student. We had a good number of group projects I had the pleasure of leading, and I learned a ton from them. I have an easier time empathizing with my boss at work, having been in similar shoes. Being a team leader means taking the well-being of others on your shoulders and being held to high standards. If you slack off, it's hard to ask the rest of the team for anything.

"My final semester, I became disillusioned with my experience. Our culture was one of intense criticism. Any time art is shown in a class, it was our practice to bring up everything wrong with it and make suggestions. Game artists do this to sharpen each other's skills, but some of the students took it too far, especially when one classmate posted a rough business card design on Facebook which criticized a fellow student's work."

Asperger's has made social interactions a challenge for Peter. "It can create tension with people, especially when I start asking questions no one would think to ask under normal circumstances, such as, 'Is humor okay with God? Should we steer this game a different direction?' Since I don't clarify what I mean by the question, this makes it hard for people to follow my line of reasoning and causes confusion.

"I tend to 'disappear' in groups of people and get interrupted when I open my mouth, due to a delay in speaking up. It might be a blessing in disguise. It's taught me to listen and observe more than talk.

"I have a goofy personality when I feel at home, and thinking in an unusual way helps me make people laugh. It helps me not disappear so much, although it can still be hard to have any part in group conversations. It doesn't help my interests are narrower than most people's . . . well, maybe not narrow, but off the beaten path."

Peter grew up dreaming about all the different kinds of video games he wanted to design. "I would try to create games using Microsoft Word. I would use the shape tools to create levels and place a circle on the level that acted as the player. This is all to say I was a creative kid growing up, and I wanted a career doing creative stuff."

Peter was finally able to make games when he downloaded Game Maker. He started creating small games; this enabled him to gain experience with coding. "My introduction to 3D art came when my friend Tyler introduced me to the still popular Roblox, a PC game where you build worlds with virtual Lego bricks that can be stretched to any length. That game got me drawing out diagrams, figuring out how to create 3D environments and vehicles with simple cubes. It matured my mind when it comes to how 3D shapes fit together. Best educational game I played."

Peter is currently designing a video game for hospital waiting rooms. "I'm working on a 3D platformer—think Super Mario 64—that has some puzzle-solving elements. It has a cool art style where we map scanned drawings onto 3D models. Its purpose is to advertise a children's hospital in a unique way and provide entertainment for kids who might be going through some hard treatments."

Hope for Employment

Parents often fear their child with autism will not have the life skills to be self-sufficient and employed. Peter is proof that the hope complex can change the outcome for people on the spectrum. But it isn't always easy, so Peter offers some tips for finding a career and being successful in it:

1. If you're passionate about a field but it looks hard to get into, just keep building your skills and hang out with people online (or, if you're lucky, in person) who do the job you want to do. Hang around the barber shop long enough, and you will get a haircut.

2. Successful, talented people are usually people who spent a ton of time developing a natural skill of theirs, but by no means did they start on top of the game. I get tired of people saying, "I can't draw," because many can draw and draw well, with a little guidance and a lot of practice.

3. Some careers are surrounded by people who say, "Yeah, nobody is talented enough for that career" (like game development), but don't give up! I grew up believing art was a "far out" job, only to meet an artist in college whose family expected him to be an artist. Now I regularly create 3D art for a living. Perspectives are all over the place due to misinformation, assumptions, or laziness.

4. We talk about being leaders a lot, but there is something to be said for being a good follower too. Managers and people in other positions of authority go through a lot of trouble to protect their underlings from office politics and put up with a ton of criticism. Give them the respect they deserve and do what you can to help.

5. Speaking of politics, stay out of those in your workplace. Don't gossip about people and instead focus on actually getting the job done. The only time to talk back at someone is to "fire a warning shot" to get their attention, but not to hurt their feelings.

Peter encourages young adults on the spectrum, "Be thankful for autism. God shines brightest in weakness, and it comes with strengths that enable us to fill certain job roles better than others would."

He adds, "Since Aspies can be workaholics, remember our work is temporary here on earth. It's not inherently bad to love working; just ensure the gain is higher than the cost. There were some projects at school I went overboard on and received little in return, other than a slightly higher grade."

While earning a college degree is one path, we must remember there are many other paths an individual can take. Technology and trade schools are also viable options and, depending on the individual, possibly better options. Degrees are still thought of as a lifelong stamp of professional competency. They tend to create a false sense of security, perpetuating the illusion that work—and the knowledge it requires—is static. It's not. My coworker Steve, a nurse with Tourette's, states, "There's a shelf life to education but not experience." Remember to lean into your son's or daughter's interests as you guide them toward gainful employment, and recognize the traditional path may not necessarily be the best.

> Many individuals with autism possess a gift for attention to detail and an intense focus, two attributes required in many professional fields.

Many young adults with Asperger's enjoy learning technology and designing computer software. The World Economic Forum predicts 65 percent of children entering primary school will end up in jobs that don't yet exist because the technology required for those careers does not yet exist.[3] This is good news since many individuals with autism possess a gift for attention to detail and an intense focus, two attributes required in many professional fields including technology and computer software design.

CLOSING THOUGHTS

A hope complex provides your child with confidence to experience life with an optimistic view of the future. You can help your children develop a hope complex by teaching self-efficacy, offering choices, seeing challenges as new opportunities, and instilling hope in Christ. As Martin Luther said, "There are times when our hope despairs; these are the times our despair must learn hope."[4]

PRAYER AND MEDITATION

Prayer

God, please develop a hope complex in my child. Hope for friendships and love. Hope for a good job and joy in work. Don't allow depression to steal our family's joy. No one whose hope is in you will ever be put to shame. My flesh and my heart may fail, but you're the strength of my heart and the source of my happiness and blessings. Shield our family with your compassion and grace. Open our eyes to your goodness and provision. When despair comes like a raging flood, make your hope overflow in our hearts by the Holy Spirit. Amen.

Meditation

> Now hope does not disappoint, because the love of God has been poured out in our hearts by the Holy Spirit who was given to us. (Romans 5:5 NKJV)

> Praise be to the God and Father of our Lord Jesus Christ! In his great mercy he has given us new birth into a living hope through the resurrection of Jesus Christ from the dead, and into an inheritance that can never perish, spoil or fade. This inheritance is kept in heaven for you, who through faith are shielded by God's power until the coming of the salvation that is ready to be revealed in the last time. (1 Peter 1:3–5)

PART 2

Therapies and Choices
That Work

Chapter 3

Prairie Dogs and Honey Badgers

It's not what we accomplish in life that matters most;
it's what we overcome.

—RON SANDISON

The wicked flee though no one pursues,
but the righteous are as bold as a lion.

—PROVERBS 28:1

IN THE SEVENTIES and eighties, before the emphasis on inclusion in the classroom, many children with autism and disabilities learned limited skills to prepare them for employment as a janitor, grocery bagger, stock clerk, dishwasher, or gas pumper. While these jobs are a perfect fit for some people, my mom was determined that would not be me.

She decided to help me refine my disabilities into beautiful gifts and talents. Autism is not something you can cure like a disease—I can't cough on you so you can get a day off work with the autism flu. However, autism can be refined.

Autism unrefined feels like walking barefoot on hot pavement and then stepping on a sharp, jagged piece of glass. It is unfiltered and inappropriate comments, rigid patterns to be followed, out-of-control stimming (that is, repetitive self-stimulatory behavior probably intended to soothe or protect), and relentless head banging, screaming, and meltdowns from overwhelming sensory stimulation. In short, it is painful.

Autism refined, on the other hand, is like walking alongside bright blue waves on a warm, sandy beach and discovering a smooth piece of glass refined by the power of the ocean. It is talents in art, science, math, or writing; it is special abilities like attention to detail, extraordinary memory capacity, or creativity necessary to develop technology.

My dad has a piece of refined glass from the ocean that measures a foot high and six inches in width. He displays the smoothly buffed gem in our house as a proud reminder of what our family has accomplished.

With God, we can all find ways to refine our jagged edges.

Prairie dogs and furry friends were stepping-stones for me being refined into the person I am today. Through my stuffed prairie dog and other animal friends, my mom taught me to socialize and to control my emotions. Learning to control my meltdowns and generalize skills were first steps to knocking off my sharp edges and essential for me gaining independence.

Before my social skills were refined, I had difficultly controlling my emotions and feelings. Learning social skills enabled me to communicate and interact with others. It took me years to understand social norms, decode body language, and handle disruption to my routines.

The social skills my parents taught me as a child established the foundation for me to attend college and have a career. My mom and dad took advantage of every opportunity. At church, my mom would remind me, "Ronnie, look people in the eyes." If I had a new friend over, she would comment, "Please, let your friend have a chance to speak also."

When I was seven years old, my mom quit her job as an art teacher and worked full-time as a "Ron teacher" using pre-ABA art and play therapy to help me learn communication and social skills—refining my autistic quirks into beautiful gifts. She believed playing and having fun with kids would break my stereotypical behavioral patterns, like lining my toys in perfect rows or collecting chocolate Easter bunnies in the refrigerator. Her hope was that being around other children would spark new interests and activities. Years later, research proves my mother's theories correct.

Dr. Pamela J. Wolfberg shares from her research in autism peer play groups that with adult guidance and peer interaction play, children with autism produced less isolated and stereotyped play and higher levels of social and cognitive play, which they maintained when adult support was withdrawn.[1]

My play activity progressed very slowly—just ask my brother Chuckie (I bit the heads off of his Star Wars figures) or my brother Steve (I used to take a pencil and rub it against the metal air vent between our rooms to create "music"). For a snack, I gnawed the joysticks of his ColecoVision video game system. Despite these struggles along the way, by interacting with my brothers and their friends, I did eventually learn how to communicate my needs using appropriate behavior.

Playing helped me to learn self-control. Katherine Reynolds Lewis, author of *The Good News About Bad Behavior*, wrote, "Games . . . help kids develop self-regulation. Both the inherent fun and the social pressure to keep a game going give children strong incentives to control their actions."[2] We all know children won't quickly play with a "bad sport" again and might even give the offender a more powerful reason to not hit or gloat or otherwise behave in a socially unacceptable way. Play becomes a place to practice skills necessary for life. I learned life skills through Prairie Pup.

Exploiting Special Interests

When I was seven years old, my mom gave me a stuffed animal for Christmas. This stuffed prairie dog quickly became my unusual special interest. In the early eighties and nineties, most boys played with G.I. Joe, Teenage Mutant Ninja Turtles, Transformers, Atari, or even a talking animatronic Teddy Ruxpin; I carried around a stuffed prairie dog named Prairie Pup.

I quickly became an expert on prairie dogs and could tell you every detail about them. My special education teacher told my parents, "Ron always carries an animal book in his right hand and Prairie Pup in his left." Prairie Pup was officially a member of the Sandison family.

My mom harnessed my special interests in prairie dogs and animals to teach me art, reading, and writing. Prairie Pup was instrumental in teaching me social skills and gaining confidence with interacting with girls. The girls in my third-grade class created cool outfits for Prairie Pup; one dressed Prairie in a cowboy costume, another as an astronaut. One even made him a Victorian dress.

My mom, Janet Sandison, shares, "One of my son's favorite activities was dictating short fictional stories about his stuffed animals and drawing illustrations. I wrote Ron's short stories in spiral notebooks. Ron drew the main characters: Chatter the Squirrel, Little Gnawing Beaver, Bouncing Bear, and Prairie Pup. I was able to teach Ron new vocabulary through writing and also helped his imagination to blossom. By watching me write, Ron was able to learn reading comprehension and memorize the spelling of words. He is a visual learner—learning best hands-on."

In fourth grade, I won the Detroit Edison Drawing contest for Oakland County by creating a poster with Prairie Pup and his furry friends building a tree fort near electrical wires. The caption on the poster stated, "Don't Become a Furry Fried Friend by Building Your Fort Near Power Lines." For the prize, Prairie and I met the captain of the Pistons basketball team, Isiah Thomas, who was later inducted into the NBA Hall of Fame.

My parents were masters at exploiting my talents, using them to help me learn self-control and to generalize information from one setting to another.

Managing Meltdowns

At the beginning of sixth grade, something horrible happened: Prairie Pup was officially expelled from the Rochester public school system. The special education department decided I was too old to be carrying a love-worn stuffed animal in desperate need of Rogaine. I felt devastated but my parents felt it was time for Prairie Pup to stay home. I needed to learn the next step in social integration.

Despite his expulsion from school, Prairie Pup still accompanies me to every speaking event. He even has a friend now: a honey badger. I purchased my first honey badger during my honeymoon in the Windy City. I saw the honey badger in a downtown storefront window. He growled at me, and I snarled back; it was love at first sight. When I purchased him, I did not realize that the stuffed animal was based on a not very appropriate YouTube video. When you press his paw, four-letter obscenities spew out in an angry lisp.

In case you were wondering, I don't bring him to my speaking engagements for fear something may brush his paw, causing him to go off before a live audience. The crowd doesn't need to think I'm giving a live demonstration of a meltdown.

Instead, I purchased a declawed stuffed honey badger from Amazon that travels with me.

I describe my meltdowns as my honey badger moments. Over the years, I've experienced many of these at home, school, and in public places. Whitney Ellenby, a disability rights attorney, gives the perfect account of a honey badger meltdown when she took her son Zack to a theater: "Autism is angry. The infuriated beast of defiance is rearing his head, snarling, writhing, biting, only I'm not trying to defeat the beast or even subdue it. I need its passion and power. It's this very passion that fuels the resistance with which I must align myself, harnessing and channeling that live energy and redirecting it toward something Zack craves but wrongly fears. Like live theater."[3]

My mom, like Whitney, used exposure therapy techniques to help me learn to regulate my sensory issues and anxiety in public places— teaching me not to fear the unknown but to trust God. Exposure therapy is a technique in behavior therapy used to help treat anxiety disorders. It involves exposing an individual to the anxiety source or its context without the intention of causing harm, but rather to help the individual overcome his or her anxiety or distress. Numerous studies have demonstrated exposure therapy's effectiveness in the treatment of disorders such as generalized anxiety disorder, social anxiety disorder, obsessive-compulsive disorder, PTSD, and specific phobias.

When I had a meltdown, there was no reasoning with me because I was overwhelmed by my emotions and sensory issues. Time alone to decompress helped me calm down. The more anxious and tired I feel, the worse my sensory processing operates. I can tolerate more noise when I am calm and alone, but less when stressed and in a crowd. The best advice is to take exposure therapy slowly, and don't give up.

My most embarrassing honey badger meltdown occurred when I was in third grade at a Cub Scouts Halloween event with Bozo the Clown. Over two hundred people were in attendance. My mom decided to have me sit front and center with the other Cub Scouts for the main event: a clown complete with red nose, white makeup, red fluffy side-hair, and a lamb sock puppet.

The poor clown knew nothing about autism and thought it would be comical to take my baseball cap, place it on another kid's head, and then place it back on my head. When the clown attempted to place the cap back on my head, I grabbed the lamb sock puppet and proceeded to repeatedly beat the clown with it. By the time I was finished, that poor clown looked like Krusty the Clown after being hit by a Mack truck.

Needless to say, I never earned my Bobcat badge. Instead, the next day, the Cub Scout leaders informed my parents, "Your son is banned from any future events. If he did that to a clown, imagine what he could do to one of our children."

Meltdowns normally decrease as your child ages, so there is hope!

Meltdowns are scary and embarrassing for both you and your child. God will get you through them—these too shall pass. In fact, meltdowns normally decrease as your child ages, so there is hope! I was in a self-contained elementary classroom until I learned to control my meltdowns and generalize information. I was in eighth grade when I mastered these two abilities and was mainstreamed.

Generalizing Skills

My special education teachers told my parents, "Ronnie is the fastest in his class to repeat back the lessons but lacks the ability to implement them." Autism caused me to lack the ability to generalize the ideas and concepts being taught or process sequences of events. Generalization is the ability to take a skill acquired in one setting and apply it to another setting. These skills are essential for employment and higher education. Along with learning to manage meltdowns, these are some of the earliest skills your child will need to refine the rough autism edges. My dad used to complain to my mom, "Ronnie is twelve, and I can't teach him how to sweep the walk. He understands how to vacuum the living room, so he should be able to sweep the walk. When I explain to him how to do it, I feel like I am speaking into the wind."

With an autistic child—or really any child— never assume that a skill taught in one situation will generalize to another situation.

With an autistic child—or really any child—never assume that a skill taught in one situation will generalize to another situation. Always give specific practice in any situation where the skill is appropriate. My mom taught me to generalize by drawing pictures of the tasks I was working on at school or home—outlining the order of sequences to accomplish it— then applying the principles I learned from the task to different settings.

In comparison, at the age of two and a half, my daughter, Makayla, has already mastered the art of generalizing. Without me knowing, she overheard my mom giving me advice.

"Ron, don't get on your soapbox with your mother-in-law when you're in Florida by talking about running for congress or sharing your political ideas."

Not heeding her advice, I found myself engaged in a heated debate with my mother-in-law when, with perfect timing, Makayla cut me off and promptly said, "Ron, off soapbox!"

My mom also taught me to generalize skills by interacting with friends and playmates. My mom would reteach the lessons I learned in the class-room through creative activities like papier-mâché or building cardboard castles. When I had friends over we read books and played educational games. My mom applied reading comprehension questions to make sure I was understanding material from school. I learned through skills of generalization to see the world from others' perspectives.

Julie Hornok shares her experience of teaching social skills to her daughter:

> We have worked consistently on social skills since Lizzie was very young. I arranged playdates with a friend from her school and a therapist in our home weekly. First, we worked on the basics like turn-taking, then moved to gross motor games, then more complex play. Thoughtfulness and being considerate is the foundation of any good friendship, so we worked on thinking from the other person's perspective and finding ways to make the other person enjoy her time in our home. We spent a lot of time planning each playdate before it actually happened to ensure it would be successful.[4]

CLOSING THOUGHTS

My mom refined my special interests in prairie dogs and animals to teach me to socialize, control my meltdowns, and generalize the skills I learned. In parenting, God will guide and direct you also and teach you how to help your child process information and handle difficult emotions. Don't give up; meltdowns will become less severe. As Philippians 1:6 states, "Being confident of this, that he who began a good work in you will carry it on to completion until the day of Christ Jesus."

PRAYER AND MEDITATION

Prayer

God, I entrust my child's future to you. Help me not to worry or be anxious. Holy Spirit, guide me with your wisdom and provide me with creative ideas to teach my child social skills and fun activities to allow him or her to enjoy life. Show me my child's gifts and use them for your glory. Help me to focus on my child's abilities. No matter what path lies in front of me, let me hear your voice behind me, saying, "This is the way; walk in it." Pour upon my family your favor and honor. In Psalm 84, you promise not to withhold good things from your children. God, I praise you for your faithfulness and love. Amen.

Meditation

> For the LORD God is a sun and shield; the LORD bestows favor and honor; no good thing does he withhold from those whose walk is blameless. LORD Almighty, blessed is the one who trusts in you. (Psalm 84:11–12)

> Start children off on the way they should go, and even when they are old they will not turn from it. (Proverbs 22:6)

Chapter 4

Therapy Adventures

Autism doesn't have to define a person. Artists with autism are like anyone else: they define themselves through hard work and individuality.

—ADRIENNE BAILON

He tends his flock like a shepherd: he gathers the lambs in his arms and carries them close to his heart; he gently leads those that have young.

—ISAIAH 40:11

LEARNING TO MANAGE meltdowns and generalize skills are obvious needs for kids on the spectrum. But sleep issues, mood disorders, and GI function issues common among kids with autism aren't always readily apparent. Setting up a team of experts to help your child thrive is critical. You can build a good team for your child by consulting friends who have children with autism, attending conferences, and contacting local autism organizations. Remember, you as a parent know your child best and you should always trust your instincts, even if it goes against what a professional says.

As you seek out therapy for your child, there are five characteristics of effective therapy to consider.

1. Effective therapy requires us to believe that change can occur with proper treatment.

Dr. Moheb Costandi, author of *Neuroplasticity*, writes, "Far from being fixed, the brain is a highly dynamic structure, which undergoes significant change, not only as it develops, but also throughout the entire lifespan."[1]

Life experience and therapy have empowered my brain to change so that it can process information more efficiently and understand social cues. Learning how my brain operates has helped me respond appropriately in making decisions, decoding body language, and feeling empathy. At the age of forty-five, my brain is still developing; I continue to experience fewer sensory issues and less social anxiety.

2. Effective therapy requires therapists who are able to connect with your child on a personal level and are able to be role models.

Metro Parent's 2017 Top Teacher, Chelsea Campbell, states, "Building connections makes kids feel special, and it leads to long-term learning gains."[2] Connecting can be as simple as the therapist taking an interest in your child's favorite movies, TV shows, toys, or video games.

The best therapists have tight boundaries with a soft heart—a perfect combination of structure and nurture. Stephanie Holmes, whose daughter has Asperger's, shares, "Boundaries with love and relationship are key for therapists and teachers working with children with autism."[3]

Finding a therapist can be difficult, but you, as the parent, can usually trust your gut. If your child isn't connecting with a therapist, consider finding a new one. The opposite is true as well. Fight like the proverbial honey badger to keep a therapist who has a good connection to your child.

3. Effective therapy is holistic, focusing on both social skills and sensory issues.

Therapists can prevent sensory overload by letting a child learn at his or her own pace. Providing periodic three-to-five-minute movement breaks is key during projects and lessons. Rachel Summers, a special education teacher, says, "Always look to the child to set the pace for learning. Look for signs of frustration, fatigue, and being overwhelmed. If you go at their speed, they'll be much more receptive to you, and you'll help them enjoy learning with you."[4]

Sonu Khosla, a developmental psychologist who works with children with autism, suggests we prioritize quality over quantity.[5] An effective therapist should keep instructions simple and concrete by giving directions one step at a time and breaking larger assignments and projects into smaller, manageable steps.

4. Effective therapy involves the whole body.

Many individuals with autism have a difficult time participating in athletics because of social anxiety and awkwardness. They may also struggle as a result of clumsiness and a lack of hand-eye coordination.

But research indicates that involvement in athletics can help a child with autism decrease their behavioral issues, depression, and anxiety just as it does for neurotypical individuals.[6] Athletics empowered me to learn coping skills to overcome many of my sensory issues and social deficits.

Let your child's natural enthusiasm guide you.

Jeremy Samson, an Australian with Asperger's and founder of Time 2 Train, shares: "I have had the honor and privilege to see some truly life-changing results, from verbal communication, to some no longer needing any further medication. From improving in coordination to a positive attitude and better overall personality, I continue to see so many successful results from a simple but effective concept in Time 2 Train Personal Training by combining physical activities with social interaction."[7]

Former MSU basketball player and autism motivational speaker Anthony Ianni shares, "There are five main benefits to athletics. When you are stressed out, shooting hoops can help relieve your anxiety. Athletics can be a cool way to make new friends. Participating in sports can build your self-esteem. Physical activities can free your mind from everything you have to do and enjoy the moment. Athletics teaches children life skills."[8]

There are five questions you can ask yourself to determine which activities your child should be involved in. Is your child naturally good at the activity? Does the activity empower your child to learn new skills? Can your child make lifelong friendships through participating? Will the activity broaden your child's interests? Is your child passionate about the activity, finding fulfillment? Let your child's natural enthusiasm guide you.

5. Effective therapy tries the unexpected.

My mom tried many different therapies and community programs to help me learn life skills. She knew that some community events and therapies would not work for me but others could produce unexpected results. One unexpected way I learned to socialize and apply lessons from speech therapy was the roller skating rink. When I was in third grade, my mom took me to the skating rink with my brother Chuckie. By roller skating I developed coordination skills and proper body movements. On the rink I felt confidence to talk to my peers without stimming and was less socially awkward—I also loved the arcade games and the greasy pizza served at the rink.

Lisa Jo Rudy, an author whose son Tom has ASD, explains another reason for parents to try the unexpected:

> When kids with autism get out into the real world, they find people, places, programs, activities, and interests they'd never have experienced in the closed box of therapies and schools. Sometimes those interests grow into volunteer opportunities or internships—in some cases, careers and relationships can result. Perhaps even more important, parents and siblings desperately need the sense of community that they are denied when children with autism are part of the family. . . .
>
> Only by getting out into the wide world can a parent see his child overcome an obstacle and rise to a challenge such as running the bases, performing on stage, or winning a merit badge.

And only by allowing a child with autism to experience the world can a parent discover a child's unexpected talent in art, music, science, or athletics.[9]

Each child with autism has unique challenges requiring a therapy program structured to meet those needs. Early intervention helps your child to socialize, communicate, and develop abilities in areas of weakness. Nine-year-old Grandy Miller is an example of the positive results that can occur from early intervention.

Grandy Miller: Splinter Skill Savant

Brittany Miller loves baseball and named her son Grandy after former Detroit Tigers' outfielder Curtis Granderson.[10] When Grandy was only three years old, Brittany noticed he had an unusual interest in fans and light switches. These were the only things that piqued his interest at the McDonald's Playland.

"I found it odd that in a room full of slides, climbing structures, and other children that Grandy refused to focus on anything else but the fan above his head. So I googled 'three-year-old obsessed with fans' and that is when I learned about autism. After reading more, I began to realize that Grandy exhibited 'red flags' like flapping, speech delay, echolalia, trouble sleeping through the night, repetitive behaviors and movements, and trouble with change in routine. The more I read about autism, the more I was convinced that my child needed to be tested."

In February 2014, a few days before his fourth birthday, Grandy received a formal diagnosis of autism. This diagnosis has since impacted every part of Brittany's life. "My greatest challenge raising a son with autism has been people's lack of understanding. People have no idea how much autism affects everything a person does right down to the things they eat! Because of this lack of knowledge, people are very quick to judge and make assumptions about my son's behavior, which puts him at risk for bullying and ridicule from strangers."

Grandy has never told his mom a lie. Everything he says is literal. He has no concept of how to make up a story or alibi. If Brittany asks him,

"What are you doing?" he will tell her what he is doing, even if it is something he knows he isn't allowed to do.

"But that also means he gets me into trouble too. Like the time I told Grandy to tell one of my friends that we were too busy to come visit, but the truth was, I just really wanted to stay home and relax. My friend asked Grandy, 'Do you want to come over to my house?' He replied, 'No, my mom told me to lie to you and tell you we are too busy, but maybe she will want to tell the truth another day.'"

Grandy is a splinter skill savant, which means that Grandy's areas of expertise splinter off into more than just one or two directions. He has the ability to quickly become an expert on anything that sparks his interests. When Grandy was three years old, he was obsessed with shapes and could identify any shape up to twelve sides and also draw them in 3D.

At age four it was microwaves; he could tell you every electronic part and its function. At age five, he was obsessed with keys. Grandy kept most of his keys stored in a box, but he also wore select favorites around his neck and clipped to his waist. His mom went to eight different hardware stores searching for miscut keys for his collection.

Once Grandy learns all that he can about his area of interest, he moves on to something else. "Last year Grandy was interested in fire alarms. He could tell you every make and model number of every fire alarm, even the vintage ones, and also identify them by their siren too. His ability to learn and store information is a true gift."

For his seventh birthday, Grandy traveled with his mom to Connecticut to visit the Honeywell fire alarm factory. This vacation was a number of firsts for Grandy. He had never been on an airplane or met so many people. "I think I was more nervous than he was about the entire trip, but Grandy did an amazing job. That trip impacted his life by giving him experiences that I alone couldn't have given him. The way he was able to communicate with other people who genuinely liked and knew about fire alarms was amazing. When you're seven years old and your main interest in life is fire alarms, it's hard to find friends your age who can relate to you."

Another special interest for Grandy is Halloween. Due to his speech delay, Grandy wasn't able to verbalize the costume he wanted until age four. After that, he always had a unique Halloween costume, including a microwave, a deck, a fire alarm, a tornado, and a haunted house. His mom says, "Every year, he challenges me by picking a costume that I have no idea how I am going to make, but every year I seem to pull it off. He definitely gets lots of extra attention and candy due to his creative and one-of-a-kind ideas. It has become a yearly tradition that my Facebook friends and family anxiously wait to see what crazy costume idea Grandy has up his sleeve every Halloween."

> While we want to pursue every therapy
> we can for our child, we must remember
> that parents need help too.

Grandy's interests change every few months. His current obsession is Apple products. He says he wants to work for Apple when he gets older, and right now he really loves watching YouTube videos about how electronics work. He knows the differences between all the iPhones and loves to experiment with how to change the settings. He also loves learning about how the internet works and what type of internet connection he needs according to the type of phone he has.

Brittany uses Grandy's special interests to help him make friends and learn. "The best way to teach Grandy is to incorporate his interests into his learning. I taught Grandy how to tell time by making a cardboard clock and using pictures of tiny microwaves on it that coincided with each number. I did the same thing when teaching him how to match pictures and colors by printing out and coloring pictures of fire alarms and having him match them. By using microwaves and fire alarms, I was able to engage him in learning. If parents, teachers, educators, and caregivers can just find a way to engage with a child with autism, then they will see the incredible amount of potential that child has."

Grandy has the ability to get people interested in what he is interested in. He was a hit when he brought a fire alarm to school for show-and-tell. Most of his peers had never touched a fire alarm before.

Making friends is still difficult for Grandy, and while Brittany encourages him to engage with others, she can only push him so far. "We attend family gatherings, birthday parties, and playdates and all of those things are practice for him when it comes to learning to make friends. I have noticed that slowly Grandy is starting to engage with other children."

Grandy is enjoying second grade at a small public school. He has a one-on-one aide with him daily in a general education classroom. Grandy's favorite time is recess because he doesn't have to work so hard focusing on a specific subject. Grandy loves playing with his friends, who are mostly girls, and he has a lot of energy, so anytime he gets to release some of that energy, he takes full advantage of it.

Parents Need Help Too

While we want to pursue every therapy we can for our child, we must remember that parents need help too. In Brittany's case, parenting Grandy has refreshed her passion for Christ. "My faith in Christ is 100 percent of the reason why I do everything in my power to educate others about autism and spread autism awareness and acceptance as much as I can. I believe that God gave me a child as special as Grandy because God knew I needed him.

"Not only did I need Grandy to make me the best mother that I can be, but God also gave me Grandy to help me find my voice again. When I was younger I used to love to write, but after my father passed away when I was sixteen, I stopped writing. I felt like I had lost that creative ability to express myself. When God gave me Grandy, he gave me a reason to find that creative ability again, a way to use my voice, to speak out, and the drive to want to make the world a better place for people with autism.

"It is through my faith in Christ that I am able to use Grandy's bad autism days—the ones where he struggles with changes in his routine, or a meltdown occurs—and not be afraid to talk about those challenges in our daily life and relate those positive and negative aspects to other people. Faith and hope are the basis of what many autism parents center their life around, because the future of our children is unknown. I live my life and parent my child with complete faith in Christ that Grandy was given to me for a reason, and while I don't always feel like I am the best parent for the job, God believes that I am, and I will do everything in my power to prove that."

Grandy teaches Brittany about life and enjoying the moment. "Grandy has taught me to notice the trees beginning to blossom, the leaves changing colors in the fall, a dandelion growing in a cement crack—he is a constant reminder that I need to slow down and enjoy all the beautiful things that God has given to me on a daily basis.

"I am in awe of the fact that Grandy looks at people and views people completely bias-free. The only thing Grandy bases his opinion on is how a person treats him. Grandy's view of the world is so simple, yet it seems so complicated to everybody else because we make our lives complicated. We move around so fast that we lose sight of how beautiful and easy the smallest things are."

Brittany encourages parents whose child is diagnosed with autism: "You are about to see the world in a way you have never seen it. You will lose some friends but gain an entire community of autism parents who, even though they just met you, will be your child's biggest fans.

"Your child's best advocate is you. Therapists and teachers aren't always right, and you know your child better than anyone.

"It's okay to cry when you think of your child's future; the unknown is very scary. Having a child with autism, you will cry more (happy and sad tears), sleep less (more opportunity to see the world), and you will create a bond with your child that the entire world will be able to see."

CLOSING THOUGHTS

Effective therapy begins with you as the parent. You know your child better than anyone else. Dig in to create methods with an expert who connects, who helps your child grow and learn. Taking a holistic, active, and creative approach can teach your child social skills and emotion regulation. As special interests change over time, you can use them to help your child learn skills for employment and independence.

PRAYER AND MEDITATION

Prayer

God, give me and my child's teachers and therapists wisdom. Enable us to connect with my child. Empower him or her to learn social skills, handle emotions, generalize concepts, and apply the things learned in therapy at home and in the community. When my child experiences meltdowns, empower us with your grace and love to overcome. With your strength, I can crush an army; with my God, I can scale walls of doubt. You, Lord, are my lamp; you turn my darkness into light. You are my help; I will sing in the shadow of your wings. Amen.

Meditation

Surely God is my help; the Lord is the one who sustains me. (Psalm 54:4)

The Lord GOD has given Me the tongue of the learned, that I should know how to speak a word in season to him who is weary. He awakens Me morning by morning, he awakens My ear to hear as the learned. (Isaiah 50:4 NKJV)

I will refresh the weary and satisfy the faint. (Jeremiah 31:25)

Chapter 5

Gifts to Be Found

*Children with autism are colorful—they are often beautiful and,
like the rainbow, they stand out.*

—ADELE DEVINE, SPECIAL NEEDS TEACHER, AUTHOR, AND SPEAKER

*Every good and perfect gift is from above, coming down
from the Father of the heavenly lights, who does not change
like shifting shadows.*

—JAMES 1:17

WHILE NATURAL INCLINATION is inherent in a person, talent is built and
cultivated, not born. It took hard work and perseverance for my gifts to
be refined. My mom invested thousands of hours using art therapy for
me to learn to read and write. My speech was so delayed, it took fourteen
years of intense speech therapy for me to learn to communicate "Th" and
"L" words. The summer of my senior year of high school, I ran more than
five hundred miles to prepare for track and cross-country.

For me to memorize over fifteen thousand Scriptures and five thousand quotes, I spent more than thirty thousand hours doing memory work. This book took me eight hundred hours to write with all the

research and interviews. Remember that developing your child's gifts will take time . . . and lots of love. Be patient.

As you seek to find these gifts and refine them, use the following tips as a guide.

1. Follow your child's interests and passions.

Be alert to what your child is interested in and gravitates toward naturally. Does your son like to build skyscrapers with Legos, or is he more likely to ride his bike to the lake and go fishing? Do you frequently find your daughter playing "veterinarian" with the cat or is she more likely to have her face in a book reading?

> Developing your child's gifts will
> take time . . . and lots of love.

Most children, both neurodivergent and neurotypical, are involved in structured activities these days, and there are many things to be learned there. But through unstructured play and exploration, children sometimes stumble on an interest that could never have come out of structured play. Give your children time on their own to discover activities that truly interest them.

Judith Newman, whose son Gus has autism, writes, "Why exactly is it Gus can't tie his shoes or use buttons, yet can play the piano with fluidity and grace? There are some things I will never understand. But it may be as simple as this: music matters and the other things don't."[1]

2. Faithfully serve others, and new gifts will be discovered.

Entering my junior year of college at Oral Roberts University, I prayed, "God, open new doors for ministry. Reveal to me opportunities to serve others with the love of Christ." During lunch a few days later, a pastoral ministry student who had speech and learning disabilities asked me, "Would you please help me with my pastoral ministry class project by participating in my small group Bible study?"

I immediately agreed and while giving his thanks, he shared, "I already asked ten other students—all of them were too busy to be part of my Bible study. I need to pass this small group ministry class to graduate."

The final chapel service of the year, this young man was awarded the ORU Overcomers Award for overcoming a severe disability and graduating with honors.

> Parents need to take notice of the things their children choose to do when they don't have to please anyone.

Perhaps your child can't study or help teach schoolwork, but they can still be kind to others. And they certainly can come with you as you reach out to your community. Perhaps they'll discover an affinity for history when you visit a nursing home, or the ability to make kids laugh when you volunteer for one of your other child's kindergarten classes. If you're willing to serve, God may very well take you somewhere just for your child.

3. Discover gifts by encouraging your children to express themselves.

Parents need to take notice of the things their children choose to do when they don't have to please anyone. Granted, giving your child the space to "do nothing" might take some planning and patience as you endure a bored child for a bit. But it's in those unplugged moments that we get to see our children's hidden gifts.

If a child loves to sit on a swing and eat a popsicle, try to discover the meaning behind swinging and eating a popsicle. Makayla loves to swing and we teach her through swinging to take turns when she goes to the park. This helps her to learn to have manners and be polite.

She loves popsicles so we use them to teach her to finish her meal before she gets a treat. We also use popsicles to teach her to offer her friends a treat when they come to visit.

Writing can be a difficult task for many with autism. Please remember that all activities that relate to writing can help move your child ahead. If he or she has an interest in short story writing, that's great writing practice, of course. But so is cartoon drawing and writing notes to put in mom's lunchbox, and making a crossword puzzle. Anything that allows your child to exercise using a pen or pencil to create words or word pictures on a page is great for moving forward with writing. And any time they can choose how and what to write or draw, they'll love it and benefit from the exercise even more.

4. Provide fun learning activities and projects.

Once you've found what your child truly enjoys, capitalize on that interest. When my mom discovered my love for animals, she subscribed to Safari Cards; each month I received a deck of twenty-four cards. These full-color cards taught me interesting facts on animals from around the world, such as where the species live, their eating habits, and predators. She also helped me create posters to share fun facts about my favorite furry friends.

If your child is interested in cars or trains, you can help his gifts develop by constructing models or visiting an automobile or railroad museum. Almost any activity or interest can be used to help a child learn.

5. Remember that gifts lead to improved communication and social interaction.

At the age of seven, Karl Birgisson had difficulty interacting with other people and speaking, but he had a real passion for Legos. On a trip to Legoland, Karl was inspired by the life-scale models and decided to build a scale model of the *Titanic*.

With the help of his parents and grandfather, plans were made. Fast-forward three years. At the age of ten, over the span of eleven months, building for more than seven hundred hours, and using fifty-six thousand Lego bricks, Karl achieved his goal. And beginning in October of 2019, Karl's twenty-six-foot-long and five-foot-tall *Titanic* replica was exhibited for a year at the Titanic Museum Attraction in Pigeon Forge, Tennessee.[2]

In an interview with Caitlin O'Kane of CBS News, Karl's dad said, "He came out of the fog and was able to communicate with people. I mean, he had to. People were coming up to him and asking, 'What are you doing?'"[3] The efforts made by Karl's family led him to a place of improved communication and social interaction through his passion. In the same way, William J. DeYonker's parents took an interest in his passions.

William J. DeYonker: Billiard Trick Shot Master Champion

William J. DeYonker experienced severe sensory issues and meltdowns leading to an autism diagnosis at age four.[4] He was behind in his speech development, unable to say complete sentences or words.

After the diagnosis, his parents researched autism, and his dad learned about Judevine School for Autism in St. Louis, Missouri. The Judevine's therapy program enabled William to develop communication and social skills.

"My mom learned about the therapy provided by Judevine back in 1996 and from there, she learned how to incorporate their teachings in practical life lessons such as placing words on multiple objects around the house and having me pronounce the words. Through this technique, I learned the name and purpose of common household items. This program also provided my mom with social stories on how kids interact with one another and helped me to interact socially."

Intense therapy was required for William to learn basic life skills. "When my mom provided therapy, she took the skills I learned in the positive reinforcement and discreet trial training sessions out into the community by having us grocery shop and then go to a toy or book store where she would buy me new books. In other words, a little bit of what my mom wants to do for the family, and a little bit of what I like to do."

Sometimes gifts are discovered in ordinary places. After watching the Disney movie *Pinocchio* at age four, William discovered a passion for the game of pool. "My interest was sparked by the scene where Pinocchio was playing pool and smoking cigars with another character on Pleasure Island. This one shot, where the cue ball hopped over one pool ball and landed on another, was the birth of my passion. Afterward, my parents took our family to my uncle's home, and I saw a pool table in the basement.

While my family and relatives were outside socializing with each other, I was busy throwing pool balls around on the table. This moment marked the beginning of my twenty-year-plus journey in pool and trick shots."

Visualization, attention to details, routines, and concentration have empowered William to perfect trick shots. "With the video reel playing in my head over the years on movies and TV shows, I was able to take that in my head and put it toward my obsession with pool. This gift enables me to visualize how the trick shot is done. My ability to concentrate and follow routines helps me to set up and continually practice trick shots for forty hours a week.

"Once I was able to focus, I accomplished amazing results in a short period of time, from being twentieth in the world rankings to first in just two and a half years."

William is currently one of the top-ranked trick shot players in the world and has won many awards.

For those wanting to become professional pool players, William offers some advice: "Be humble when competing against other trick shot artists, and understand that you are only doing your shots for your own points. If you try to show that you're better than the other players, you'll never achieve success."

William's toughest obstacle to overcome was his social skills. "The greatest challenge I experienced as a high school teenager was engaging with my peers. I found it easier to engage with people at least ten years older than me, because they understood how to interact with people and what's really important in life."

William discovered inspiration in Philippians 4:6, "Do not be anxious about anything." This verse helped him overcome his fear of trying new things and gave him confidence in unfamiliar social surroundings, such as college, to make new friends.

Faith in Christ was key for William's success. "From my perspective, Christ certainly helped me overcome a lot of obstacles in life. When I was young, my folks took me to Northridge Church every Sunday for over ten years. This church taught me to apply Jesus's teachings to my life and how to be a disciple.

"Previously, I was in a pretty dark and depressed place until I discovered at fifteen I have autism. After that, I slowly came to understand how Jesus had lifted my spirits when I was young and learned how to stop regressing to my old and reclusive lifestyle in my early teenage years. I was baptized at sixteen. I realized Jesus had a purpose for my life and would use my autism for his glory."

After graduating from high school, William attended college. While at school, life both at college and at home became stressful.

"I was dealing with stress from the amount of work I had to do and learn while trying to excel and be a high-honors graduate. I learned to push aside my home life issues and keep focused on the projects I needed to complete. This time prepared me for managing my adult life and adapting to stressful situations. When things get stressful in the future, I know how to handle them because of those chaotic college years.

"I pray daily, even during my darkest seasons, about how God made my life a blessing from all of the encounters I've experienced since I was diagnosed. I couldn't be more proud; the Lord has helped me with new lifestyle changes and enabled me to adjust to life more easily."

William is now employed full-time as the brand ambassador for Centria Autism, speaking at schools and organizations and sharing the great benefits and unique abilities people with autism provide to our world.

William encourages parents to "discover your child's gifts by trying different activities he enjoys until you discover his niche—work at developing it into a career or social learning experience. Do research on activities relating to your child's interests and give him chances to pursue it. Believe God has given your child gifts and pray he will teach you to refine them."

William advises young adults with autism to "keep being who you are. There isn't another person like you and there never will be. Focus on your talents and keep learning how you can brighten people's lives. If you can't find someone who brightens up your day, then be that person who brightens up everyone's day."

CLOSING THOUGHTS

Therapy, early intervention, discovering a gift, and faith in God have empowered William to lead a productive life and develop into a world-class trick shot pool player. Since he began competing professionally in 2013, he has won master championships in Oklahoma, appeared in ESPN's Trick Shot Magic event, and traveled to China for the world championships. While your child might not travel the world and win championships like William has, he or she also has amazing gifts to be found—discover those talents by taking an interest in what your child loves.

PRAYER AND MEDITATION

Prayer

God, open my eyes to the gifts you have given my child. Teach me by your Holy Spirit to cultivate and refine those talents. Bring teachers and mentors into my child's life to develop those gifts for communication and social interaction. Bestow favor and honor upon my child's life. Empower my child to use those gifts for your glory and to advance your kingdom. Amen.

Meditation

> The kingdom of heaven is like treasure hidden in a field. When a man found it, he hid it again, and then in his joy went and sold all he had and bought that field.
>
> Again, the kingdom of heaven is like a merchant looking for fine pearls. When he found one of great value, he went away and sold everything he had and bought it. (Matthew 13:44–46)

Thanks be to God for his indescribable gift! (2 Corinthians 9:15)

Chapter 6

Painted Butterfly

When you are worried or anxious, look to Jesus.
—Kimberly Dixon, poet

*Therefore be imitators of God as dear children. And walk in love,
as Christ also has loved us and given Himself for us, an offering
and a sacrifice to God for a sweet-smelling aroma.*
—Ephesians 5:1–2 (nkjv)

When I was diagnosed with autism, my mom chose to trust God and focus on my abilities. She prayed for the Holy Spirit to guide and direct her in teaching me social skills. Through prayer, the Holy Spirit revealed to her that I was a visual learner and art was the best way to teach me, which is one of the many excellent ways to reach autistic children.

While I am completely verbal now, it is estimated that as many as 25 percent of individuals living with autism spectrum disorders are non-verbal. For these individuals, keyboarding speech, poetry, and other forms of writing can be a perfect mode for communication. As Psalm 19:3–4 says, "They have no speech, they use no words; no sound is heard from them. Yet their voice goes out into all the earth, their words to the ends of the world."

Virginia G. Breen, the mother of Elizabeth, a nonverbal poet with autism, writes: "Just as a poem stubbornly refuses to allow itself to be summarized, so it is with Elizabeth. She can't be summarized by a diagnosis, a label, or a first or second impression. To know her is to take the time to understand her on her own terms, at her own pace, in her own words. Like art and music, poetry invites us to come to it on its own pace, in its own words. So for Elizabeth poetry is the perfect vehicle, because it can't be summarized or put in a box."[1]

> The most life-changing art is
> often the result of struggle.

It's no secret that having autism or parenting a child on the spectrum is difficult. But we also know that the most life-changing art is often the result of struggle. Kathie Maximovich, the mother of Nicholas, a young adult nonverbal artist with autism, shares, "Breaking boundaries is one of the ways we experience life to its fullest potential. That is what Nicholas's artwork has done for him. Expression through abstract artwork is his way of communication without words. The beautiful part is, everyone sees and experiences something different when they look at his work."[2]

For me, art allowed my learning to progress. It was slow, though, causing me to have frequent meltdowns from frustration. Through it all my family loved me unconditionally and believed God would not only use my creativity and art for his glory, but that I was a beautiful work of art myself. As Psalm 139:13–14 says, "You made all the delicate, inner parts of my body and knit me together in my mother's womb. Thank you for making me so wonderfully complex! Your workmanship is marvelous— how well I know it" (NLT). Dr. Lamar Hardwick, a pastor with Asperger's, gives great insight to who we all are in Christ: "With God there is no need for a second edition of me. Autism won't keep me from becoming a better husband or father or pastor. Autism and all the struggles that come with it may at times keep me from loud rooms and long meetings, but it won't keep me from my best because I am exactly who I am supposed to be. I was born with all of the potential to become the most courageous and creative version of me that God always intended me."[3]

N. T. Wright said, "Those in whom the Spirit comes to live are God's new Temple. They are, individually and corporately, places where heaven and earth meet."[4] It doesn't matter that my mind works differently; I am a place where heaven and earth meet—I am exactly who God created me to be. Through art and nature, I am able to express the Lord's goodness, communicating his grace in my drawings of animals.

> When we are unable to communicate
> with words, God can still use our gifts of
> creativity to express his grace and love.

Kimberly Dixon, a nonverbal poet, is a testimony of God's goodness by displaying Christ's beauty in art, writing, and poetry. When we are unable to communicate with words, God can still use our gifts of creativity to express his grace and love. Augustine of Hippo said, "Our rewards in heaven are a result of God's crowning His own gifts."[5]

Kimberly Dixon: Spiritual Poetry and Artwork

On April 29, 1985, Jim and Marilyn Dixon were filled with joy as God blessed their family with a beautiful red-headed girl.[6] She was healthy and active—full of life. She was progressing normally, even gaining some skills early.

At seven weeks old, Kimberly had a minor reaction to a medication she was taking. But around four months old, her parents began to notice some cramping spells; their family doctor believed that they were symptoms of colic because they were more frequent when Kimberly was constipated.

When she was six months old, Kimberly received a second dose of the medication and her reaction was dramatic. She passed out, turned gray, and was rushed to the hospital. By the time the family doctor saw Kimberly, she appeared fine, and the X-rays revealed her lungs and heart to be normal. In the days that followed, Kimberly became more listless, began having severe cramping spells, and appeared to stop progressing developmentally. Very concerned, the Dixons took their daughter to a developmental pediatrician who referred them to a pediatric neurologist who diagnosed her with infantile spasms, a rare form of epilepsy.

Jim and Marilyn share: "Kimberly's allergic reaction to the medication began our thirty-one-year journey of seizures, hospital stays, therapies, and doctor appointments from San Diego to Philadelphia. Throughout our journey, we learned to trust Christ and rely on his strength."

Jim and Marilyn had Kimberly enrolled in an infant-parent program. The infantile spasms continued. Her progress was slow, but she learned to walk and later to read. However, Kimberly was nonverbal and seemed to be in her own world, which led to an autism diagnosis by age ten.

These spasms progressed into other types of seizures, including tonic-clonic seizures and drop seizures that threw her to the ground. In an attempt to help Kimberly overcome her seizures, her parents tried anticonvulsants, supplements, brain surgery, a VNS implant, chiropractic treatments, diets, and many other therapies.

Finally in 1992, when Kim was six, a communications breakthrough occurred after viewing a program on Prime Time Live about facilitated communication. Marilyn created a keyboard from poster board and began teaching Kim to type words using a hand support technique. Kim quickly learned to type short sentences and express her thoughts. By age eight, she was writing creative stories; by age ten, she was writing inspiring poetry. As time progressed, Kimberly was able to type her words with only light elbow support on communication boards and devices, iPods, and computers.

Kimberly wrote over one hundred poems and won many awards for her poetry. In 2013, Kimberly and Marilyn published a book of poetry and art titled *Under the Silence Is Me—How It Feels to Be Nonverbal.* Some key themes of Kimberly's writing and art include the wonder of creation, birds, animals, God's glory, Christ's love, and experiencing life. Thomas à Kempis, author of *The Imitation of Christ*, writes, "There is no creature, regardless of its apparent insignificance, that fails to show us something of God's goodness."[7] In her first poem, "Friends Role of Love," Kimberly shares her desire for friendship.

Friends dance across my life,
Answering my cries and strife,
I begin singing in my heart,
And naming all the friends I cart.
Opening vast oceans of love,
Being friends is like wearing a glove.
My friends hold me tight,
And keep me from fright.
Joy fills my life when friends are here;
I pray my friends will always be near.

Kimberly's greatest struggle in life was her frequent seizures; she had thousands of them and captures the terror of having one in her poem titled "Seizure."

Moaning in the night
Really frightening dreams
Feel angry inside
Loony noises in my head
Flashes of light
Awful pain in my brain
These are seizures.

Autism caused Kimberly to experience fear and anxiety. She discovered comfort in Christ and her favorite Bible verse was 2 Timothy 1:7, "For God has not given us a spirit of fear, but of power and of love and of a sound mind" (NKJV). Through poetry, Kimberly expressed her innermost thoughts and, most importantly, her love for God.

My Wonderful Savior

Great is my God
Full of mercy and hope.
Great is the Lord
Who is bringing me joy.
Great is the King
Who is king of my heart.
Great is my Master
Who loves me the most.

Poetry empowered Kimberly to find peace in a world that can be overwhelming and scary.

Roping the Moon

Suddenly you turned around and . . .
The people roped the moon,
And the moon slowly came to earth.
Men came to look for the moon that night;
But the Sky was free of the light of the moon.

Sounds of sadness echoed in the night.
Lonely and afraid, little children cried.
As the darkness filled the sky,
Young teens could not drive.
Old ones fell in the Street as they crossed;
Dear souls hurt and lost.

Mothers gave their children hugs
Calming their fears with love.
Dads helped their teens drive home,
And girl scouts aided the lost and alone.

Suddenly you turned around and . . .
The yellow moon had returned,
Bringing its light back to earth.

When you saw the glow, you wondered—
Had this all been real,
Or had time stood still?

Through poetry Kimberly shared her love of nature and animals. Kimberly rode horses weekly as a part of her therapy. Horse riding became a sport where she could feel at peace and experience a sense of normalcy. Throughout her life, Kimberly remained steadfast in her faith in Christ and desired to live a life that brought glory to God.

On April 25, 2016, Kimberly wrote her final poem. Earlier that month, Kimberly and her family had gone to Butterfly Days at the Emily Ann Theater in Wimberley, Texas, which was started twenty years ago by the Rolling family when they lost their daughter in a car accident. Each year at Butterfly Days, thousands of butterflies are released in memory of loved ones who have died.

When Kimberly released her butterflies, one of them landed on her leg and stayed with her for forty-five minutes until her parents released it in a butterfly tent on the property.

Kimberly was so moved by this experience that she wrote "The Painted Butterfly," describing Christ's power to transform our weaknesses into his glory. She then put the poem into a beautiful painting. Her mother, Marilyn, shares, "It was as if Kimberly knew her life in heaven was soon to begin."[8]

Two months later, Kimberly had a drop seizure, falling and hitting her head. She suffered two brain bleeds and went into a coma, awaking into eternal life six days later.

The Painted Butterfly
In the trap of a cocoon, a caterpillar is waiting.
All his energy is stored inside.
As he gives up his old life,
His new beginning is soon to arrive.

Instant change will open a new life;
Death of the old must happen first.

Popular caterpillar will go away
To be replaced by a creature so fine.

When the beautiful butterfly is ready,
He pushes his way outside his cocoon,
Gains his strength and flies away.
Painted butterfly has now joined the world.

CLOSING THOUGHTS

Art is a great tool to help children with autism learn social skills and communicate their ideas. Through art, your child's creativity and faith can blossom. You can teach your child to express his or her feelings and emotions. Art can also provide relief from anxiety and sensory issues. You might even find it enjoyable to sit down and create with your child.

PRAYER AND MEDITATION

Prayer

As the masterful potter, Father, shape our lives and create a beautiful design. You are the builder and hold the blueprints of my child's life. Let me trust you to complete the good work you've begun. God, you are my provider and my strength, and you are my child's provider and strength. Reveal the gifts you've given my child, and show me how to refine those gifts for your kingdom. Amen.

Meditation

But now, O Lord, You are our Father; we are the clay, and You our potter; and all we are the work of Your hand. (Isaiah 64:8 NKJV)

This is the word that came to Jeremiah from the Lord: "Go down to the potter's house, and there I will give you my message." So

I went down to the potter's house, and I saw him working at the wheel. But the pot he was shaping from the clay was marred in his hands; so the potter formed it into another pot, shaping it as seemed best to him. (Jeremiah 18:1–4)

Chapter 7

Fierce Love and Art

Art washes away from the soul the dust of everyday life.

—PABLO PICASSO

*A man's gift makes room for him, and brings him
before great men.*

—PROVERBS 18:16 (NKJV)

WHEN CONVENTIONAL FORMS of therapies like applied behavior analysis (ABA), speech, and occupational seem to produce limited results, visual art therapy may be the path to your child learning to communicate and socialize. I was reminded of this on March 22, 2017, when I opened a letter from Dr. Laurence A. Becker, founder of Creative Learning Environments and the producer of *With Eyes Wide Open*, a documentary film about the life and wax oil crayon art of Richard Wawro, an autistic savant from Edinburgh, Scotland.

Dear Ron, I was surprised by the synchronicity of discovering your book, *A Parent's Guide to Autism: Practical Advice. Biblical Wisdom* this past weekend while we were in Houston filming

Grant Manier and his mother, Julie, for my new documentary film, *Fierce Love and Art*. While the cinematographer, Ron Zimmerman, was filming Grant at work, I was sitting nearby and happened to look at the titles of several books in his bookcase. I picked out your book, began reading the endorsements inside. . . . I would welcome an opportunity to meet with you or talk on the phone.[1]

The next day, Dr. Laurence and I talked for over an hour. I loved hearing about his new documentary *Fierce Love and Art*. As he spoke, I desired to be one of his featured artists. This documentary film shares stories of autistic savants and prodigies whose parents used art, music, or poetry to help their child blossom creatively, learn social skills, and experience life.

Children showed more motivation, paid closer attention, and remembered what they learned more easily when the arts were integrated into the curriculum.

Grant Manier, whom I interviewed while writing *A Parent's Guide to Autism*, is an example in the film of the power of using creative outlets to transform a child. As a toddler Grant obsessively tore pieces of paper. His mother, Julie, patiently nurtured Grant's love for brightly colored tissue paper. He learned gradually to arrange the torn bits into beautiful wildlife artwork. Many of his large collages contain as many as 3,500 pieces of repurposed calendars, magazines, and gold paper. Grant went on to found the nonprofit organization Grant's Eco-Art.

Since starting Grant's Eco-Art, he has raised more than $250,000 for many charitable organizations to help those with autism, epilepsy, Down syndrome, and other disabilities. Grant's 38" by 48" eco-original of J. J. Watt's Touchdown, created by using over 15,000 pieces of recycled puzzles, raised $3,000 for J. J. Watt's Charity Foundation.

Grant developed social skills and confidence through his artwork. He often says, "It's not what you can't do; it's what you can that makes you more."

In May 2017, Dr. Laurence emailed that my family was chosen to be part of the documentary along with seven other families. After they filmed Dr. Darold Treffert, a world-renowned expert on savants and prodigies in Wisconsin, I would be the final stop on their 2,500-mile road trip.

Dr. Laurence and Ron Zimmerman filmed me at my parents' house in Rochester Hills, Michigan. Earlier in the day, they interviewed my parents. My mom proudly displayed all my artwork for them. I shared in the documentary how my mom quit her job as an art teacher and became a full-time "Ron teacher." On May 13, 2018, I was in Austin, Texas, for the premier of *Fierce Love and Art* and met Grant Manier and his mom, Julie Coy, along with the rest of the artists.

Art and Learning

A Johns Hopkins University School of Education 2009 research study reported that children showed more motivation, paid closer attention, and remembered what they learned more easily when the arts were integrated into the curriculum. Cognitively, emotionally, and culturally, the arts can connect people more deeply to the world and open them to new perspectives. It's clear that arts education adds value to children on more levels than simply increased academic performance.[2]

Claire Draycot, a special education teacher, encourages parents: "Some young autistic children may struggle with their fine motor skills, for which the simple act of guiding crayons over paper can render a huge improvement. However, as well as honing their motor skills, making drawings allows autistic children to communicate thoughts and feelings they may otherwise struggle to express. Viewing a child's drawing opens a window into interests, preoccupations and emotions which may go unregarded in a child with ASD, who does not communicate these things in a conventional manner."[3]

Art therapy can open up myriad opportunities to an individual with autism who has artistic talent. It can also create unique opportunities for

personal bonding, improvements in ability to imagine, thinking symbol-
ically, recognizing and responding to facial expressions, managing sensory issues, and developing fine motor skills.[4]
Art develops a willingness to explore what has not existed before. Art
teaches risk-taking, learning from mistakes, and understanding that
there could be more possibilities than are readily apparent. Creativity
also develops curiosity and passion for deeper knowledge.[5]

Painting, writing, and music can also help your child develop a healthy self-esteem.

Painting, writing, and music can also help your child develop a healthy
self-esteem. The arts support the expression of complex feelings for children who don't necessarily have the words for these complex ideas. This
helps kids feel better understood and helps them understand others when
viewing others' artwork. The arts support personal meaning in life, finding personal joy, and spreading joy to others.[6]

Haley Moss demonstrates the power of using art to develop a child's
self-esteem.[7] As an infant, Haley cried continuously, and she was nonverbal until age three. In preschool, Haley could arrange complex jigsaw
puzzles, but lacked the social skills to interact with her classmates. When
Haley was diagnosed with autism, specialists warned her parents that she
"would be lucky if she has one friend, graduates from high school, and
receives a driver's license." Her parents were told not to expect too much
from her. After her diagnosis, some parents wouldn't let their kids play
with Haley because they thought her condition was contagious.

At nine years old, Haley was obsessed with Harry Potter. Her mom,
Sherry, used Haley's obsession to help her understand her diagnosis: "Much like Potter, you are also different from your peers and have
magical powers. Beside an extraordinary memory, autism has given
you strengths with computers skills, artistic talents, and a gift for writing. Different is not a bad thing. It is just different. And different can be
extraordinary."

At thirteen, Haley spoke on a panel at the Autism Society of America Conference. After her presentation, she was encouraged and inspired to write a book to help middle school students on the autism spectrum. Over the next two years, she wrote a 160-page book, *Middle School: The Stuff Nobody Tells You About.*

Haley shares, "I'm not the best with social stuff, and in middle school, I wasn't into talking about boys and makeup and parties like the other girls my age were. I also lacked social common sense, but I learned from my mistakes."

When Haley was young, Sherry helped her daughter learn through floor-time play and other activities while encouraging Haley's interests. She worked tirelessly with Haley, trying different methods until she found strategies that worked. Haley's mom used a structured schedule of activities to help Haley develop her social skills. Haley says, "My playtime with peers was very organized. When other kids came over for playdates, my mom had a set time for snacks, games and activities, and for the kids to return home. I felt more relaxed making friends by having a routine schedule I could follow because I knew what to expect."

Haley experienced severe difficulty in social interactions, but she excelled at art. Haley had always enjoyed creating artwork and began to receive recognition for it when she was thirteen. She explains, "Drawing helped calm me down and escape from the social drama of school as well as stress." Haley paints anime-style characters with acrylic on canvas. Her artwork has been compared to world-renowned Brazilian neo-pop artist Romero Britto. Haley's work has been featured in galleries through-out South Florida. Some of her original paintings were sold for thousands at an auction to benefit the University of Miami and Nova Southeastern University's Center for Autism and Related Disabilities.

Haley is only twenty-five and has already graduated from the University of Florida with a BS in psychology and a BA in criminology, then she went on to graduate from law school at the University of Miami. She is the first practicing lawyer with autism in the state of Florida, working as an associate with a law firm in Coral Gables.

Haley shares, "I want to see a world where people with disabilities achieving things is a norm rather than an exception. It isn't a surprise when you see an autistic person practicing law or doing something amazing in the world."

Art develops our whole brain, boosting our self-confidence and ability to express feelings while also freeing us from anxiety. Art also strengthens focus and increases attention, develops hand-eye coordination, requires practice and strategic thinking, and involves interacting with the material world through different tools and art mediums. Haley is a model of art's ability to transform our self-image and help us see the world from a new perspective.

Art and Social Interactions

Communication in relationships can be complicated. But for people on the autism spectrum, often there aren't enough words to express the feelings, emotions, and ideas necessary to grow a relationship.

When I was a freshman in high school, my first girlfriend and I broke up, and she refused to talk with me (to be fair, I poured a drink from Wendy's on her head).

But then I wrote her this poem.

First Girl to Ever Love Me

She was the first girl to ever love me; some guys have been around this world, but none could've had a girl as lovely as her. She had this inner beauty that drove me insane with love every day. As we kissed I felt the heat of her magical lips. Then came that fateful day—as the trees lost their leaves so she lost her love for me.

I still love her true to this day. I wish I could look one more time into her mystical eyes and see that paradise on earth. But until that day, I hope and pray that she'll forgive me for all the things I said and did.

For I was just a boy who did not know what love was until she came along my way. Oh, how lucky I was then when she was mine and only mine.

After reading my poem, she called my house, and I apologized for my childish behavior. We remained friends throughout high school. Poetry restored our broken friendship.

The art of poetry reopened the door to our relationship. True, it was no longer romantic, but we developed a real friendship. Poetry allowed me to essentially create myself in a new way that communicated well with a friend. In a way, poetry was like magic that day; it helped to heal two hearts that had been broken.

Transformational Power of Art

Seth Chwast, another artist, was diagnosed with autism at age two. He was profoundly autistic and nonverbal, and though in his mid-thirties now, he is still unable to cross the street by himself or put away his art supplies. Debra, his mother and the author of *An Unexpected Life*, shares: "At eighteen, Seth had a formal vocational evaluation that determined he was best suited to a career in dry mopping. There we were in the dusty little office where Seth had just completed a three-day evaluation to determine his potential for employment. All that work, all those therapies, all the hours that we and others had devoted to him—with all that he could do, the result was dry mopping? I said, I would die first."[8]

A dramatic change came in 2003 when, at age twenty, Seth took a four-week art class at the Cleveland Museum of Art. Seth, who rarely speaks, began describing his world in paint. He displayed an innate ability to mix colors and create amazing works of art that reflect his vision of his world and the world around him. And over time, Seth's artwork has attained international notoriety. Debra now has local college students who are art majors mentor Seth three to five days a week. Seth helps teach the college students about autism and art while the students provide Seth with companionship.

Debra states, "Seth paints day and night. He is autistic and that's just a small piece of who he is. He is also kind, gentle, loving, sensitive, funny, and creative. Seth is unstoppable and has created over 850 paintings. When he paints, he knows exactly what he wants. He is amazing, and he is as certain about paint as he is lost in the real world. I encourage all parents, never give up—you have no idea what your child is going to accomplish."

Seth desires to change the world and states, "Seth's art will make people feel all better. My art will make people feel calm and comfort and tranquil."[9] Debra and Seth travel around the world selling his paintings; his artwork has been displayed in galleries in New York, Gallops Island, and France.

Art as Business

Art is big business. At the core of the multibillion-dollar film and video game industry are artists creating images and stories. Every commercial product is artistically designed, from chairs to cars, space stations to iPods. In 2017, a Leonardo Da Vinci painting sold for $450 million.[10] Young adults on the spectrum who struggle with conventional employment and feel out of sync in an office environment may discover art as the perfect career.

Eight Ways to Spark Your Child's Interest in Art

My mom discovered eight ways to help cultivate my love of art that you can also use with your child. These activities will help you and your creativity too!

1. *Start early.* Pablo Picasso said, "Every child is an artist. The problem is how to remain an artist once he grows up."[11] Art can start with a few crayon scribbles, but when a child likes the feeling, he will keep doing it, and drawing and creating can develop into a lifelong skill. Children will develop a sense of well-being as they do artwork, as well as a feeling of security.

2. *Make art fun and relatable.* If your child likes a particular character, animal, or object, such as Thomas the Train, Pokémon, or spaceships, have her use those in her artwork. Since I loved squirrels, bears, and prairie dogs, my artwork always included these furry creatures.

3. *Keep art supplies close by, but not too close.* Purchase crayons, markers, and watercolor paints for your child. Keep an easel set up somewhere for the kids to access easily. Just a word of caution, though: if your child is four, like my daughter, Makayla, remember to keep the

drawing supplies out of reach. I learned this lesson the hard way. As I settled in to watch the Super Bowl one evening, I noticed Makayla had drawn a rainbow on our TV with markers and crayons. Oops.

4. *Give your child freedom to be creative with their artwork.* In a 1929 interview, Albert Einstein said, "Imagination is more important than knowledge. Knowledge is limited. Imagination encircles the world."[12] Let your child's imagination soar and take him wherever he wants to go. Allow ample time and space to create. Then keep a portfolio, either hard copy or digital, of your child's artwork. It's not just a neat memento for you as a parent, but it can help your child gauge just how far they have progressed artistically. Children, like adults, love to experience progress and feel motivated by this.

5. *Set aside time for art.* Create a regular time slot for your children to work on art. It could be a little every day, once or twice a week, or on the weekends. Remember to give your child your undivided attention during art time.

6. *Look into art lessons, classes, or programs.* Libraries have many art programs, and most communities offer community education classes for children. Looking online can be a great way to find local art programs.

7. *Plan trips to art museums and galleries.* Every major city in the world has some kind of art museum network. Since I grew up near Detroit, to spark my interest my mom took me to the Detroit Art Institute and the annual Art & Apples Festival, a fine arts fair with exhibitors from across the United States.

8. *Praise your child's artwork.* Kids' artwork, no matter what it looks like, is always wonderful! Let your child know how much you love it! Don't criticize her art or tell her how to do things, and above all, don't micromanage creativity. As G. K. Chesterton said, "There are no rules of architecture for a castle in the clouds."[13]

CLOSING THOUGHTS

Art can empower your child to communicate, learn social and problem-solving skills, develop fine motor abilities, and have a healthy self-esteem.

Creativity helps other skills to develop and hidden talents to emerge. It's been said that Aristotle believed that the aim of art is to represent not the outward appearance of things, but their inward significance.

PRAYER AND MEDITATION

Prayer

God, develop my child's creativity and gifts. Let your beauty and grace be expressed through my child's artwork and talents. Holy Spirit, reveal to me ways to spark new interests in life and discover fun activities we can enjoy together as a family. As my child matures, bring loving mentors, creative artists, and wise teachers who can inspire and help refine those gifts. Empower my child to reach their full potential. Thank you for creating beautiful things for our enjoyment and enabling us to create beautiful things to honor you. Amen.

Meditation

The heavens declare the glory of God; the skies proclaim the work of his hands. (Psalm 19:1)

He has filled them with skill to do all kinds of work as engravers, designers, embroiderers in blue, purple and scarlet yarn and fine linen, and weavers—all of them skilled workers and designers. (Exodus 35:35)

Chapter 8

Excellent Choices

Autism is not something you fix;
it's something you adjust to.

—RON SANDISON

He will rescue the poor when they cry to him; he will help the
oppressed, who have no one to defend them.

—PSALM 72:12 (NLT)

HAVE YOU EVER noticed how weather forecasters offer the most obvious advice on a hot summer day? "It's a hot one today, so if you're out in the sun, drink plenty of water and wear a hat." Or my all-time favorite tip: "With 98-degree scorching heat, many people will be swimming today, so if you don't know how to swim, don't go in the deep end." I remember a newscaster last Fourth of July reminding viewers, "If you decide to shoot fireworks, make sure you do it outside with adult supervision."

My mom received a lot of similar, unsolicited, and utterly useless advice because of my behavioral and sensory issues. A speech therapist once told her, "If your son would only try harder and practice his 'Th' and 'L' sounds, people would be able to understand him."

"Why don't you get Ronnie on a sugar-free and dye-free diet? Then he won't have meltdowns during recess," a fellow mother suggested.

A school counselor recommended, "If you take away his love-worn stuffed prairie dog, he will socialize better with his peers and make friends."

There are times when you need to shrug off advice.

"Why don't you talk with the pastor about parenting? He has four well-behaved sons," a concerned Sunday school teacher counseled.

Listen

Diane Dokko Kim, whose son Jeremy has autism, offers some illuminating insight on the power of listening to someone, rather than offering empty words of encouragement:

> The first thing I try to do, before offering any kind of sharing, is to listen. Listen has the same letters as silent. I remember vividly when we first received the stunning diagnosis, well-meaning friends, family and church members tried to say things to encourage us like, "God only gives special kids to special parents. It's because he knew you could handle it." I knew they meant well but it only stung an already bleeding heart.
>
> In contrast, wise and compassionate friends simply listened. They received and validated how I felt, regardless of how raw, unruly, and conflicted my emotions were. They were willing to show up and hold an emotional barf bag for me. They let me fill it, without judgment or admonishment to be more spiritual or "Just trust God!"[1]

As a parent of a child with autism, I am sure you have also received unwanted advice in the most awkward of places, such as the grocery store or at work. While the advice is meant to be helpful, it comes largely from a place of ignorance about autism. Advice like, "If you just put your child on a gluten-free diet, he will be cured of autism" or "ABA therapy worked wonders for my daughter; you should do the same" only isolates us further, causing feelings of resentment.

Decisions, Decisions

There are times when you need to shrug off advice. But sometimes there really are things that need to be explored and decided on. Do we try a new therapy? Would this medicine help? Do we need to change schools? While we've hopefully learned not to allow fear to paralyze us, how is a parent to move forward and know they've made the best choices? There are certainly times when parents of kids on the spectrum feel overwhelmed.

Galatians 5:25 encourages us to "keep in step with the Spirit." But what does keeping in step with the Holy Spirit look like, and how do we do it? I offer five pieces of advice that helped my parents and that now help me. As you apply these principles, the Holy Spirit will give you wisdom for raising your children and peace in your daily decision making.

1. Stay cool, and keep your peace of mind.

Karla Akins, parent of twin sons with autism and author of *A Pair of Miracles*, describes the Holy Spirit's guidance and power in parenting:

> When you don't know which therapy to use, or whether the doctor's advice is the right choice for your child, *be still*, and wait for [the Holy Spirit] to guide you and show you which way to go.
>
> When you have been on the phone with insurance for five hours straight and still have no answers, *be still*, pray, and give the battle to the Lord.
>
> When your child is out of control, you can be in control by *being still* and staying calm. Not easy, I know, but again, with him, you can.
>
> This isn't a license to throw up your arms and be passive. Stillness is an action. By being still you are actively obeying him and listening for his voice. He has a plan. He's got this. He

knows what's best and he will not fail to show you which way to go. He is fighting for you, not against you. He has your best interest at heart, and that means he has the best interest of your child at heart too.[2]

It's easy to become frustrated with parents and teachers who keep giving you unwanted advice. Or how about trying to stay calm while handling your child's meltdowns and behavioral issues? How often do we lash out at other people when we feel overwhelmed? But Ephesians 4:26 states, "In your anger do not sin."

Note that the verse does *not* say, "Never get angry." There are some healthy ways to express your anger, but don't let it cross over the line into sin. Here are just a few ideas for healthy ways to process anger. If you feel out of control in the moment, give yourself a time-out to regain your composure. Do something physical, such as walking or dancing. Talk about how you feel with someone you trust and who is a good listener. Try to pinpoint the exact reasons why you feel angry, so you can consider different strategies for the next time you encounter the situation.

Pray for God to show you how to release your anger without an emotional breakdown and for the peace of Christ to rest upon you. As Colossians 3:15 says, "Let the peace of Christ rule in your hearts, since as members of one body you were called to peace. And be thankful."

2. Walk in the Spirit, not the flesh.

Being calm is the first step in making wise decisions. But how do you actually choose? How do you walk forward?

Galatians 5:16–18 advises, "So I say, walk by the Spirit, and you will not gratify the desires of the flesh. For the flesh desires what is contrary to the Spirit, and the Spirit what is contrary to the flesh. They are in conflict with each other, so that you are not to do whatever you want. But if you are led by the Spirit, you are not under the law."

Operating by the flesh is what gets us in trouble—looking for what makes my life easy, giving in to my flashes of uncontrolled anger, holding on to unforgiveness. Anything that focuses on me and grasps for my rights or comforts might mean I'm operating in the flesh. It all comes down to motives. Am I reacting selfishly? Am I self-focused? Are my thoughts focused on me and my comfort and my rights?

When you and I can sincerely ask, with our whole heart, what's best for others and what honors God, then we are operating by the Spirit. That doesn't mean that we think nothing of ourselves. It simply means that our primary focus is outside of ourselves. The interesting thing is that when we start living less for ourselves and more for God and others, we suddenly find life a whole lot more enjoyable.

3. Expect God to prune you.

Jesus said, "Every branch in Me that does not bear fruit He takes away; and every branch that bears fruit He prunes, that it may bear more fruit" (John 15:2 NKJV).

We know we are becoming more Christlike as our life displays more "love, joy, peace, patience, kindness, goodness, faithfulness, gentleness, and self-control"—the nine fruits of the Spirit (Galatians 5:22–23 NLT). But what's a little harder to get our arms around is that God's pruning causes us to produce the fruit of the Spirit.

I experienced pruning during my junior year of high school. To grow spiritually I had to cease hanging out with my friends who were partying and not serving God. During this season, I began to study God's Word and quit swearing. At the end of the pruning, I had new friends and a greater knowledge of God's Word along with a love for people with disabilities.

When a child melts down, we can choose to grow patience. When a coworker says something unkind, we have an opportunity to grow self-control. When it looks like all hope is lost, faithfulness has an opportunity to grow.

Of course it isn't easy to take difficult circumstances and learn to use them to bear fruit, and that's where walking in the Spirit is so important. Keeping in communication with God will point out areas that need pruning, and open our hearts to God's pruning, so we can bear the fruit of the Spirit.

4. Take breaks when you need them.

A simple definition of *burnout* is doing too much, with too little, for too long. Terry Pagliei shares, "Learn to understand when you are beginning to feel overwhelmed, and find ways to manage your stress. If you are stressed, your ability to be what your child needs will be impaired. Caring for yourself will be very beneficial to yourself and your child."[3]

If you're feeling stressed, schedule a break for yourself. This might mean calling someone to watch your children for a few hours, saying no to extra responsibilities (even that call for help in the kids' wing at church), skipping scrubbing the kitchen for a day, going for a walk outside, or playing the piano. You know best what helps you to feel refreshed and what is possible in your circumstance. Do that. Your child needs you to have enough space in your life to care for them. And you certainly can't bear fruit if you're wilting from self-neglect.

Psalm 143:10 reminds us to ask the following of God: "Teach me to do your will, for you are my God; may your good Spirit lead me on level ground." You will run your best race when you aren't running uphill carrying a load of stress but instead are on the level ground God intends for you.

5. See each day as a fresh start to live by the Spirit.

Ethan Hirschberg, a seventeen-year-old with autism, wrote the following on his blog, *The Journey Through Autism*:

> No matter what happened the previous day, my mom always starts the morning off as a new day. I have been very physically aggressive at times, as well as saying some very disrespectful or hurtful things. I used to have meltdowns that would last for hours and hours. I sometimes have consequences that go into the new day, but my mom always wipes the slate clean in her head. She doesn't take things personally. This helps me to move on from what happened instead of having to keep talking about it or feel upset about it over and over again. This also helps to keep our relationship strong![4]

Miranda Keskes, a mother of a nine-year-old son with autism, shares her struggles with maintaining her cool in stressful situations:

It's hard to keep my emotions from elevating when my son's do. When I'm especially tired or frustrated, I have my own form of a meltdown. However, allowing my son to see me get overwhelmed helps him understand he's not alone in controlling his emotions. It's the repair work we do together after our meltdowns that is so important. We talk about what happened, we learn from our struggles, and we forgive ourselves so that we can try again, allowing ourselves the grace of a fresh start. Our relationship continues to strengthen through our shared struggles.[5]

I also have learned to see each day as a new beginning. Autism causes my mind to experience an overwhelming fear of the future, so I pray each morning, "Holy Spirit, let your peace guide my life. Empower me to look beyond my failures and experience your grace each day."

Barbara, the mother of Rachel Barcellona, demonstrates the fruits of staying in the Spirit rather than the flesh.

Rachel Barcellona: The Ability Beyond Disabilities

In infancy, Rachel Barcellona achieved her developmental milestones at a regular pace, speaking at nine months.[6] But when Rachel was two years old, her mom, Barbara, noticed Rachel did not enjoy playing with her classmates at preschool and isolated herself in the back corner. She was extremely sensitive to noises and was terrified of fire drills. Barbara remained calm and refused to be frustrated, despite her daughter's diagnosis with autism at age three.

Recalling her early days with autism, Rachel shares, "I can remember not being able to put enough pressure on a crayon to make a mark on a paper! Buttons, zippers, and snaps were a nightmare! It was very difficult to hold objects and jump and skip. I went through several years of physical therapy, speech and language therapy, and occupational therapy which helped a lot. I still cannot ride a bike, although I haven't tried a three wheeler, and I am not able to drive. I passed my learner's permit for driving, but because of epilepsy and seizures, I cannot get my license . . . yet! I joke with my parents that I am waiting for the Google car that drives itself!"

Rachel's seizures can be life threatening. At age eleven, during a particularly violent seizure, Rachel experienced cardiac arrest. Barbara, a nurse practitioner, responded quickly and saved her daughter's life.

A lack of social skills, awkwardness, and epilepsy caused Rachel at age thirteen to have a low self-image, self-injury behaviors, and suicidal thoughts. In middle school, Rachel attended a Christian school where she felt rejected by her peers and school administration. Rachel's love of heavy metal music, unusual social behavior, and swearing caused the students and principal to refer to her as "the devil."

Rachel shares, "I was tormented by bullies. I once made a friend with a stray dog, and a boy who loved to tease me killed the dog in front of me. The dog was my only friend."

"Our challenges should never limit our dreams."

Because of Rachel's autism diagnosis, many people told Barbara she would not be successful. Barbara chose to walk in the Spirit and bear fruits of perseverance by not allowing the naysayers to steal her joy. With the help of her parents, though, Rachel was determined to prove the skeptics wrong. Barbara encouraged her daughter to take drama classes, participate in beauty pageants, develop her singing talent, and build her self-esteem by volunteering as a Big Sister.

Rachel does not allow autism or unwelcome "advice" to hinder her from accomplishing her dreams. She focuses on what God has called her to do and chooses to walk in the Spirit. And it shows. She graduated from high school with a 3.6 GPA and went on to study theater and music education at St. Petersburg College. Utilizing her talents, she was crowned Miss Florida International in 2016, Miss Southeast International in 2017, and Miss Manatee River in 2019. She then became an international spokesperson for the Center for Autism and Related Disabilities (CARD-USF). Currently, she is enrolled at the University of South Florida, majoring in International Studies, with the dream of becoming a global ambassador to the United Nations.

In 2019, twenty-two-year-old Rachel spoke before the UN about ending stereotypes surrounding autism, sang at Madison Square Garden for the third time, and was the first person with autism to compete in the Miss Florida pageant.

Rachel desires to continue her education by earning a doctorate in special education and then opening a school to help children with disabilities.

She encourages young people with autism and their parents with these words: "I believe that autism is not an excuse for anything. Everyone has a mountain to climb and autism has not been my mountain; it has been my opportunity for victory. However, I did not always believe that. People always told me that I could not do much of anything and that I would never be successful, but my parents never let those people bring me down. My mother always encouraged me to participate in modeling to boost my confidence. . . . We all have dreams in life and we all have challenges in life, but our challenges should never limit our dreams."

Rachel and her parents chose to walk in step with the Holy Spirit, and in doing so found a path full of fulfillment and joy.

CLOSING THOUGHTS

Don't allow unwanted parental advice to hinder you from receiving sound advice, such as, "Never take your child to a doctor whose office plants are dead." Walking with the Spirit enables you to keep a positive attitude when facing challenging circumstances. Pray for the Holy Spirit to give you discernment and wisdom in parenting. As the apostle Paul said, "And this is my prayer: that your love may abound more and more in knowledge and depth of insight" (Philippians 1:9).

PRAYER AND MEDITATION

Prayer

God, please help me to receive advice with humility and the discernment of the Holy Spirit. Don't allow my heart to become callous with a judgmental attitude but let it remain pure before Jesus. When I'm faced with difficult decisions, I trust you to show me the way to go. Surround me with your peace and love. Amen.

Meditation

> You turned my wailing into dancing; you removed my sackcloth and clothed me with joy. (Psalm 30:11)

> Trust in the LORD with all your heart and lean not on your own understanding; in all your ways submit to him, and he will make your paths straight. (Proverbs 3:5–6)

Chapter 9

Fear Not

Fear will keep you up all night, but faith makes one fine pillow.
—Philip Gulley, Quaker pastor and author

*This is what the Lord says to you: "Do not be afraid or
discouraged because of this vast army. For the battle is
not yours, but God's."*
—2 Chronicles 20:15

Life is filled with fear and anxiety, ranging from fear of natural disasters
to worry over sickness, from the anxiety of unexpected bills to making the
best choices for our children. One of my greatest fears is the dentist. I
experience severe anxiety waiting in the lobby, worrying about how many
cavities the dentist will uncover from my candy-binging habits—or worse,
maybe they'll say I need a root canal. I also fear routine physical examina-
tions because I hate having my blood drawn. However, all these fears are
minuscule compared to the concern parents have for their children.

In the midst of your fears and storms, Christ calls out, "Fear not! I love
you; I am concerned for you and your family." When the disciples were in
a small boat in the Sea of Galilee, battling the raging waves, Jesus called

out to them, "Be of good cheer! It is I; do not be afraid" (Matthew 14:27 NKJV). Probably not exactly what Peter expected as they struggled.

> Peter responded, "Lord, if it is you, command me to come to you on the water."
>
> "Come," Jesus replied.
>
> Peter immediately jumped out of the boat and walked on water toward Jesus, but when he heard the sound of the wind, he became terrified, took his eyes off Christ, and began to sink.
>
> Descending into the darkness, Peter cried out, "Lord, save me!"
>
> Jesus lovingly reached out his hand and lifted Peter from the water.
>
> "You of little faith," Jesus said. "Why did you doubt?" (author's paraphrase based on Matthew 14:28–31)

Like Peter, in the midst of our storms in life—public meltdowns, therapy schedules, IEP meetings, taking care of the needs of our families—we also experience fear and doubt. *How will I ever get through all of this? Why me? Lord, I'm sinking.*

Laura Kasbar, whose twins Ana and Max have autism, shares how fear led her to hope:

> I had a nervous breakdown. I couldn't sleep. I couldn't remember anything. I cried all night. But somehow, I knew I had to push through. Those experts telling me Max belonged in an institution was the best thing they could have said to me. It drove me into action. As parents, we need to have a very healthy combination of fear and hope to move forward. If we don't have hope, we stop, and if we don't have fear, we don't bother. I had plenty of fear, and I was determined to find hope. . . .
>
> The most unexpected gift in this journey is that instead of me taking care of Max for his entire life, he already takes care of me. He is willing to help me all the time with his little brother and makes my life easier every day. As an extra added benefit, he even engages with us now more than the TV.[1]

It is easy to say don't be afraid, but trust isn't something easy to actually practice . . . especially as the parent of a child on the spectrum. In my experience, there are seven ways we can trust God in the midst of the autism storms that sometimes surround us.

1. Remember God is more powerful than your fears or your child's behavioral issues.

When Peter focused on the storm and wind—outward circumstances— he took his eyes off Jesus and was unable to walk on water. He feared a storm raging beyond his control, took his eyes off his Lord, and, as a result, began sinking. And some of us are sinking too. Instead of fearing that which you cannot control, keep your focus on God, sharing with him your fears and concerns through prayer. Be honest with God; ask him for his strength, grace, and guidance. God is our source of strength in the midst of our fears and anxiety.

Theologian and professor Henri Nouwen writes: "When I trust deeply that today God is truly with me and holds me safe in a divine embrace, guiding every one of my steps I can let go of my anxious need to know how tomorrow will look, or what will happen next month or next year. I can be fully where I am and pay attention to the many signs of God's love within me and around me."[2]

2. Don't be ruled by emotions.

Even though it is difficult, try not to be shaken or ruled by your emotions. Instead, put your trust in God that things will work out as they should. As Isaiah 26:3–4 says, "You will keep in perfect peace those whose minds are steadfast, because they trust in you. Trust in the LORD forever, for the LORD, the LORD himself, is the Rock eternal." Anne Moore Burnett, whose son has autism, writes, "A positive attitude enables you to look at what appears to be an impossible situation and find alternative ways to make it work."[3]

3. Keep a faith journal of God moments.

Isaiah 7:9 says, "If you do not stand firm in your faith, you will not stand at all." A faith journal helps you stand firm in faith by reminding you that

God is in control and working in your family's life. Keep a record of God's presence in those seemingly random moments that are masterfully woven together by him to create a beautiful work of art: a knowing smile from a fellow parent as you walk down the grocery aisle with your child, a stranger paying for your coffee, or an unexpected snow day. There is beauty in these simple moments, but they are easy to forget. When you write them down, you can go back when you're struggling and be reminded of the good things God brings into your everyday life—the God moments.

4. Face your fears head-on by making lists.

Accepting your fears rather than ignoring them can be a very powerful tool. To help alleviate the stress that accompanies my fears, I tackle them head-on by making a two-column list. In column one, I record my fears and the dates I experience them. In column two, I record the aftermath of each fear. This helps me understand if my fear was founded or not; in most cases, it was not.

Fear Factor List

Flying Frontier Airlines (11/2/18)—fear of being bumped from my flight from Michigan to Austin, Texas.	I didn't get bumped from my flight to Texas or flight home to Michigan (11/5/18)—I also had a good conversation with the passenger sitting next to me. This passenger even purchased from Amazon a copy of my book *A Parent's Guide to Autism* for his brother, who has a son with autism. Also, the wing of the airplane had a cool picture of a mountain goat.
Going to the dentist (11/19/18)—fear having a mouth full of cavities and decaying teeth, costing me thousands of dollars.	I went to the dentist—I only needed a deep cleaning to remove bacteria, calcium, and debris that collected under my gum line and had one filling replaced (12/3/18)—I didn't have to refinance anything to pay the dentist's bill.

Annual end-of-the-year job performance review (1/3/19)—fear nursing supervisor will complain about my autism quirks and lack of job performance standard.	My supervisor met with me for my annual job performance (1/3/19)—he only had compliments and praise for my performance.
My first colonoscopy (9/5/19)—fear of colon cancer.	I had five small polyps removed for biopsy during my colonoscopy (9/12/19)—results revealed the polyps were noncancerous.

Maritza A. Molis, author of *Autism in Our Home*, has a son with autism, Jaiden, and suggests: "Make a list of what brings you joy and what you are most grateful for. Whatever it is that has been bothering you, write it on a paper, and if you can help it, great, if not, lay all of your problems at the feet of God. It is hard at times. Trust me; I know. I have learned to envision myself putting it on my back porch and saying, 'Okay, Lord, there it is. I am giving all of it to you believing you will see me through. Okay, bye-bye.'"[4]

5. Pray for Christ to set you free from fear as he transforms you into his image.

There's nothing inherently wrong with being afraid. Even Jesus experienced fear. He was "deeply distressed and troubled" (Mark 14:33) in the garden of Gethsemane on his journey to the cross and the resurrection.

Years of raising a child with autism can make you feel chained by fear of the future. The apostle Paul wrote, "Now the Lord is the Spirit, and where the Spirit of the Lord is, there is freedom. And we all, who with unveiled faces contemplate the Lord's glory, are being transformed into his image with ever-increasing glory, which comes from the Lord, who is the Spirit" (2 Corinthians 3:17–18).

The Greek word for "transform" in verse 18 means an outward change from an inward transformation, such as a caterpillar turning into a beautiful butterfly.

The apostle Paul used "transform" in a way that demonstrates that God is the divine source of our transformation; it's not something we do in our own strength. As the Spirit sets us free from fear, he transforms our fear into faith. As we pray, the chains of fear are broken, and we are transformed "into his image with ever-increasing glory."

6. Allow yourself to rest as our ever-present God takes charge.

Jesus walked on water to his disciples in the midst of the storm. Isaiah 43:1–2 says, "Fear not, for I have redeemed you; I have called you by your name; you are Mine. When you pass through the waters, I will be with you; and through the rivers, they shall not overflow you. When you walk through the fire, you shall not be burned, nor shall the flame scorch you" (NKJV).

> When we understand God's unconditional love for us and that he is in control of everything, fear will no longer motivate our decisions in life.

Amy Mason, author of *Bible Promises for Parents of Special Needs Children*, shares: "Spiritual amnesia makes me forget that I am God's child. I am the beneficiary of God's kindness and his wisdom and understanding. I also forgot that my storm is a puny gust of wind compared with the strength and power of my heavenly Father. A word from his lips can transform the swirling seas to calm waters."[5]

When we understand God's unconditional love for us and that he is in control of everything, fear will no longer motivate our decisions in life. It is a concept many of us know in our heads, but don't truly understand. First John 4:18–19 states, "There is no fear in love. But perfect love drives out fear, because fear has to do with punishment. The one who fears is not made perfect in love. We love because he first loved us."

Envision God's perfect love focused on you and your child, and rest in that love.

7. Speak words of faith to your child.

Proverbs 18:21 says, "The tongue has the power of life and death, and those who love it will eat its fruit." That means how we speak to our children can harm our children or comfort and encourage them. And we all know that fear sometimes causes us to do or say things we wouldn't normally.

Janet Lintala, author of *The Un-Prescription for Autism*, writes, "Get rid of yelling and dump the sarcasm. Many ASD children cannot interpret the meaning of a raised voice and sarcasm and it just agitates them further. Their mood will mirror yours. Your house will be calmer if you modulate your voice."[6]

Amanda Grace LaMunyon, a twenty-four-year-old Christian artist from Oklahoma with Asperger's, demonstrates the transforming power of faith in Christ to overcome life's storms.

Amanda LaMunyon: Adventures with Faith and Art

As a young child, Amanda struggled with school and peer interactions.[7] Even though she began reading at age four, in kindergarten, Amanda was easily distracted, couldn't sit still in class, doodled on papers, and had difficulty comprehending the rules of the classroom. Sherry, Amanda's mom, shares, "First grade was overwhelming for her. She continually got in trouble at school—her little spirit was really hurting."

In 2003, at age eight, she was diagnosed with Asperger's. This diagnosis helped Amanda understand how her mind processes information. "Focusing was an issue for me," Amanda says. "My mind would be going a mile a minute so it tended to be difficult focusing on one thing unless I was very interested in it. At school, I kind of felt out of place. Socially, I always felt like I was a stranger."

Amanda had a hidden, congenital savant ability for art locked inside her brain; at age eight, this gift would transform her life and give her something to latch on to when she felt afraid and out of control. Sherry hired an art teacher to help Amanda express her frustration in a healthy way. After her first private art lesson, Sherry's worries were relieved as she entered the room and saw Amanda and the teacher both smiling and dripping in paint. Amanda proudly showed her mom the watermelon paintings she had made. The teacher said to Sherry, "I think this girl can paint!"

"When I put a paintbrush in my hand for the first time, I instantly felt my life change," Amanda says. "I could finally focus without getting distracted, and my paintings helped me convey everything I had difficulty expressing."

Through painting, Amanda was able to overcome social awkwardness, and develop friendships and self-confidence. "Learning I had Asperger's helped me come to terms with my different brain wiring and made me all the more passionate to exercise my talents with painting. I always wanted my artwork to be enjoyed, but hearing about how many others have Asperger's like me, I wanted my artwork to mean something and help other people."

Sherry enrolled Amanda in various classes to help her learn social skills and display her talents. Everyone who saw Amanda's paintings was amazed by her attention to detail and creativity. By age twelve, her artwork was on display in New York City art galleries and received international exposure. Art has empowered Amanda to overcome her fear, become more outgoing, and speak publicly on autism and the challenges she experiences. Amanda discovered her ability to help others when she gave a painting to a former teacher who had cancer and later learned it had greatly lifted the teacher's spirits in her last days.

On April 2, 2008, Amanda, at age twelve, read her poem, "A Little Secret," written about her journey with Asperger's, at the United Nations for World Autism Awareness Day in New York.

She looks like any other little girl.
But she holds a secret you might never suspect.
There is something about her.
She often talks about Ancient Egypt and nothing else,
Even if you don't want to hear about it.
She is very well meaning, but frequently misunderstood.
Some say she is a "little professor."
She knows a lot about what interests her.

Her clothes bother her a lot.

Just a little tag might feel like sand paper.

Food needs to taste and smell right or she won't eat it.

She thinks she can't go a week without ice cream.

Noise in the lunchroom really gets to be confusing, and She
wants to say Be Quiet!!!!

Light . . . . is 100 times brighter to her. Oh, what a world she
lives in.

What is this little secret she holds?

It's called Asperger's Syndrome, a high-functioning form of
autism.

Many people are suspected of having it.

Einstein, Michelangelo.

1 out of every 59 children will be diagnosed with autism this
year.

How do I know so much about Asperger's Syndrome?

I know because I have it.

Some say it is a disability.

But I am a girl with dreams.

I will take what God has given me.

Along with the challenge and use it.

To fulfill the purpose He has for me.

Let me say to you, if you know someone who seems a little different Look for something good.

It will be there. It may be just "a little secret" waiting to be told.

A dream waiting to unfold.[8]

"The biggest challenge I have is overcoming the way others view me
because I have autism," Amanda says. "However, I have learned that I am
just the way God intended me to be. I am perfectly imperfect. The Bible
says, 'God knew me before I was in the womb and that I am perfectly and

wonderfully made.' I have to remind myself of this fact from time to time. There have been many challenges with dealing with the world around me, though many of them I have learned to deal with.

"When I was very young, I used to throw myself on the floor and scream, and no one could figure out what I was screaming about. It was almost always in a public place. When I was older and could explain, I told them that I was afraid of heights. That made no sense because it was never when we were up high. I finally could explain that it wasn't looking down that was bothering me. It was looking up. When I looked up, I felt like I was falling up. The doctor said it was because I would lose my balance. So after that discovery, my parents gave me big hats and sunglasses to wear when we were in that kind of situation. I'm doing much better with that now.

"I still get nervous and feel out of place in some social situations, especially when I'm with people I am not familiar with. Big groups seem to be the hardest. The older I get, I try to find ways to cope with different situations. I sometimes struggle with being independent, or I should say *wanting* to be independent."

Art helps Amanda enjoy life. "It is relaxing for me to paint, and it is a way to express myself when I can't find the words. Before anyone knew I had the gift of painting, I was always getting in trouble at school, and I think people viewed me as a troublemaker. But when I started painting, I became known more as the girl who could paint. This helped give me confidence in who I was."

Faith is an important part of Amanda's life and helps her understand who she really is and why she is the way she is. "I accepted Christ as my Savior when I was very young. I know God gave me gifts for a reason. I want to use my life and my gift to encourage others that God gives everyone a gift. The biggest gift anyone can have is the gift of God's Son, Jesus. I haven't always understood what this really means. But I am beginning to understand that it isn't what I do or don't do that makes me a Christian. It is what God has already done. The fact that no one is perfect and yet God loves us anyway is a wonderful thing. Christ says that in our weaknesses we will know him and his strength.

"In today's society and culture, it can be challenging to believe God is in control. Sometimes I question why certain things happen the way they do and why I do some of the things I have done. Faith is believing something you cannot see and yet still believe. But even in these times, God is growing my faith. I am learning to be patient! Being an adult is challenging."

Amanda encourages us to "never give up. Be patient and try to listen to those who love you and want to help you. Believe God made you just the way you are and loves you. People with autism are like everyone else. We have hopes and dreams. We may seem different but we truly are not less."

In fact, Amanda has enjoyed experiences most people only dream of—like being featured on *The Today Show*. "I was extremely surprised and honored to know that I was invited to be on *The Today Show* with Megyn Kelly. There are many artists with autism who are so talented, and I was very humbled. The experience was uplifting for me."

> Life is challenging for individuals with
> autism with severe depression and
> anxiety, but we can discover peace by
> following Christ's plan for our lives.

As Amanda thinks about her future goals, she shares, "I have always enjoyed art, so I want to use art in some way. I also love children. I am learning that God has given me other abilities too and I want to be versatile. I want to always be an advocate for the awareness of autism and the abilities people have with autism."

Amanda reminded me of the importance of trusting Christ and not allowing our fears to hold us back. Life is challenging for individuals with autism with severe depression and anxiety, but we can discover peace by following Christ's plan for our lives. In our weaknesses, God manifests his strength.

CLOSING THOUGHTS

We will experience storms and terror of the unknown. Everyone does; it's part of life. As we look back over these seasons of uncertainty, we will see the most growth occurred when we kept our eyes on Jesus, placing our trust in God to save us and carry us through.

PRAYER AND MEDITATION

Prayer

God, meet me in all my fears and anxieties. You are my light in darkness. You lift me up when I am sinking. I will keep my thoughts focused on you. Let me find rest in your goodness and grace. Lord, you promise to never forsake me, so I can say with confidence, "The Lord is my helper—whom shall I fear?" Amen.

Meditation

So do not fear, for I am with you; do not be dismayed, for I am your God. I will strengthen you and help you; I will uphold you with my righteous right hand. (Isaiah 41:10)

These things I have spoken to you, that in Me you may have peace. In the world you will have tribulation; but be of good cheer, I have overcome the world. (John 16:33 NKJV)

Chapter 10

That's Life

A Christian who is not armed or prepared to suffer is like a
soldier who goes to battle unarmed.

—JOHN BEVERE, *BREAKING INTIMIDATION*

Carry each other's burdens, and in this way
you will fulfill the law of Christ.

—GALATIANS 6:2

WHEN I THINK of the perfect family, I realize it's a myth, as I learned from my friend John. John's family seemed perfect—five brothers, all star athletes and exceptionally bright; a dad who was a successful entrepreneur; and a dynamic, beautiful mom loved by everyone.

Everything shattered in 2005, when his younger brother Paul was in a severe car accident and the youngest, Jack, died. The perfect family was shaken; his parents divorced, and Paul developed mental health issues. I was reminded that nobody gets through this broken world unbroken.

All of us experience hardship. As Job 5:7 says, "Yet man is born to

---

This chapter is dedicated to the memory of my father-in-law, Bob Boswell.

trouble as surely as sparks fly upward." My neighbor shared a humorous story about raising his daughter. He had just purchased a sixty-inch flat-screen TV. A week later, his six-year-old daughter decided to clean the new TV with a cocktail creation of bleach, Comet, gasoline, and window cleaner, destroying his new entertainment system. Not all hardships are equal in magnitude, but they can be painful, nonetheless.

Building a healing community can help us get through. Myroslaw and Maria Tataryn, parents of a daughter with Rett syndrome, a rare neurological disorder, and coauthors of *Discovering Trinity in Disability*, share the importance of brokenness in community: "The true human community is built upon the One whose body was broken for the sake of love. To be in relationship with God, then, is to recognize one's brokenness and so to share in the community of solidarity created by Christ's Cross. The notion of 'unbrokenness,' then, is merely an idea that varies according to context and relationship, just as having a disability may or may not be disabling for an individual."[1]

We live in an imperfect world filled with grief and suffering. As parents of children with autism or other special needs, we need a healing community of friends, coworkers, and professionals for support and help. Needing extra help from friends and neighbors does not make us weak; rather, it empowers us to stand strong and thrive in the midst of crisis and uncertainty.

Professor Thomas E. Reynolds, author of *Vulnerable Communion*, has a fourteen-year-old son with Asperger's and shares:

> We inhabit the world in particular places of welcome, dwelling in homes that on a local scale mediate a sense of being at home in the larger world. We are like thirsty travelers craving the nourishing replenishments of a home that receives us with cool water. And the wellspring of such welcome is not something we discover alone. Home is a dwelling place marked by the presence of other people. It is a communal place of orientation in which we fit comfortably, grow roots, and reside safely. Its welcome is constituted by relationships formed within a specific social network that nurtures familiarity and preserves trust. We desire to

be recognized and accepted, woven together with others. . . . We feel at home in the world by dwelling with others.[2]

My daughter, Makayla, loves attending events at the public library with her grandma. She sings with the other children and enjoys a sense of belonging, but for people with autism, attending public events or movies can be a nightmare. Fortunately, sensory-friendly events and movies are now more readily available; attending these events with other families who understand the isolation of autism can supply the emotional support you need to survive.

> Community is meant to give you a place
> to be heard and understood by those who
> know . . . because they've been there.

Connecting with other families who are traveling the autism journey creates a valuable community. In that community both neurotypical family members and those on the spectrum engage with new ideas and opinions they never would have encountered in isolation. A community brings activity and opportunities to embrace new ideas and stretch your creative thinking. But most of all, community is meant to give you a place to be heard and understood by those who know . . . because they've been there.

And when we expand our communities to include other helpers, we can find support and healing. Healing communities are formed by people who empathize with your pain and help you deal with your grief. Your healing community may consist of counselors, pastors, and other parents with special needs children. There are five benefits of being a part of a healing community that I have found to be true.

1. A healing community can help you keep pace with life.

As we all know, life is filled with unexpected circumstances and unforeseen challenges, especially when raising a child. Three days after my father-in-law passed, my wife and I flew to Florida to be with her family.

My sister-in-law Heather is an avid runner, and I decided to go for an early 7 a.m. run with her and my brother-in-law, Charlie. With my college and high school track star days far behind me, I was having difficulty keeping up. I felt exhausted, using all my energy in an attempt to maintain pace, but still dragging a good thirty feet behind their speedy pace. Realizing I was struggling, Heather and Charlie readjusted their pace so I could keep up for the rest of the suburban marathon.

Having a child with autism and special needs can make you feel much the same—out of sync, unable to keep up with life's many demands. However, a healing community of friends can restore a feeling of order and rhythm in your life. Forty-plus hours a week of ABA therapy, not to mention speech and occupational therapy, can cause you to lose balance. How do you find time to care for your other children, work, fix dinner, mow the grass, clean the house, or get the car oil changed?

A community can provide you with a network of support and encouragement. Relatives and friends can help by allowing you to rest when the pace is faster than you can run.

You need to be honest and open, letting your family and friends know you are reaching, or have already reached, your breaking point. Many of your friends and neighbors likely want to help, but they may not know how to ask and feel awkward doing so. Let people know simple ways they can help you and your family. Maybe your mother-in-law has offered to bring dinner once a week. Let her. Or perhaps you ask for a grocery delivery service membership as a gift so you can do all your shopping from your phone while at appointments. Or you let your friend network know that your other children would benefit from playdates at least once a week—preferably on the same day—so you can catch your breath.

Your spouse may work full-time and be away from the home; let him or her also know your struggles. Raising a special needs child can feel like a sprint, but the truth is, it's a marathon; learn to pace yourself. Run when you can and need to, but give yourself permission to walk sometimes too.

2. A healing community can alleviate fears.

Caring for a child with autism can be isolating, lonely, and scary. There's a real fear of the unknown: Will he ever wear a Halloween costume? Will she go to prom? Will he grow savvy enough to deal with other people without being taken advantage of? Will she ever be able to live on her own? Will I ever know what it feels like to have an "empty nest"? And all of these questions and fears bubble to the surface because our child isn't developing typically. With our child's meltdowns and other surprising behaviors, invitations to social events eventually dry up, and we can begin to feel embarrassed, misunderstood, and alone, and one day we find ourselves isolated from other people.

A community of fellow parents further along on the autism journey can help bring you comfort and advice, and break the isolation. These parents understand your fears and can lead you to available resources. They provide emotional support and escape from the shame and guilt that accompanies autism. Deborah Reber shares:

> Many of us turn to Facebook for comfort, connecting with a handful of parenting support groups filled with strangers bonded by our shared experience of navigating what sometimes feels like an endless onslaught of obstacles. And when we have those *really* bad days—the ones where we fear we won't survive one more meltdown or shaming look—we reach out in desperation, wanting more than anything to know that we're not alone, that we're not crazy . . . that it will get better. We share lurid details of a public tantrum or an embarrassing showdown with a teacher or a frustrating conversation with an unsympathetic relative, and cry tears of gratitude for the virtual hugs and words of support that come streaming in.[3]

3. A healing community can bring joy in the midst of sorrow.

The apostle Paul wrote, "Rejoice with those who rejoice; mourn with those who mourn" (Romans 12:15). Having a friend by your side makes life's painful moments more bearable. A well-timed quip or just a listening ear can encourage someone who's struggling.

Human interaction is rarely more important than in times of grief. Small things like a gentle touch can bring healing. Sometimes the best thing we can do is provide a hug or a comforting hand on the back. I have difficulty understanding social norms due to autism, but I learned quickly from Clinical Pastoral Education to provide a comforting hand to the back with a silent prayer when ministering to a family who has experienced a tragic death.

Job 2:13 says, "Then they sat on the ground with [Job] for seven days and seven nights. No one said a word to him, because they saw how great his suffering was."

4. A healing community can create a sense of belonging.

Autism can cause you to lose a sense of normalcy because of your child's meltdowns or inappropriate comments in public. For some people, it creates a fear of leaving the house, but meeting with other parents with children on the spectrum can help you regain connection with life. Marina Sarris from Interactive Autism Network at the Kennedy Krieger Institute states, "Managing meltdowns, wrangling with teachers about special education needs, avoiding sights or sounds that overload your child's senses, and drives to therapists or doctors. And that's just what Monday looks like. Moms and dads do all this while sleep-deprived."[4] All of these challenges break normalcy. But when you find a place of belonging, you find people who struggle as you struggle, and who can help you discover peace, self-esteem, and ways to cope with emotions and life's stressors.

Angela Gachassin writes: "Some of the best reference information is the other parents sitting in the waiting room while your children are in therapy. Speaking with other parents of autistic children is such a learning experience. We were like our own little family, all reaching for the same goal, to help our children progress. We shared stories with laughter and sometimes with tears. At the same time, you feel a connection with other people who are experiencing your emotions, concerns, hopes, and dreams."[5]

5. A healing community can provide the strength to keep going.

Raising a child with autism requires perseverance and dedication. When Charles Spurgeon taught about all of the animals who made it onto Noah's ark, he reminds us that not just the fastest animals got on board, but the perseverance of snails helped them reach the ark as well.[6] Micah 7:8 declares, "When I fall, I will arise; when I sit in darkness, the LORD will be a light to me" (NKJV). As we fall and get back up again, there are times that our healing community is the light that the Lord sends to us.

In parenting a child with unique needs, there will be times of darkness: trying to choose the right school, dealing with behavioral issues, or being wait-listed for therapy programs. God promises to be our light in the darkness. Don't give up—your family needs you.

Pastor Andrew and Rachel Wilson, parents of two children with special needs and authors of *The Life We Never Expected*, share, "When you're tired, everything in your life is affected: your physical health, your emotional well-being, your ability to process things mentally, and (because it is often the easiest thing to neglect) your spiritual growth."[7] Having a community around you can empower you for the long journey ahead. In fact, Scripture tells us that other believers are to be so close that "if one member suffers, all the members suffer with it; or if one member is honored, all the members rejoice with it" (1 Corinthians 12:26 NKJV).

Community can empower you to keep going through prayer, encouragement, acceptance, and fellowship. Our prayers do not magically cause problems to disappear as if they have entered the Bermuda Triangle, but they can open our eyes to the invisible God and his power and wisdom. Mother Teresa said, "Prayer feeds the soul—as blood is to the body, prayer is to the soul—and it brings you closer to God."[8]

Pastor Chad Lewis writes: "Prayer in its most basic form has a beautiful childlike quality about it. It requires nothing more than a pouring out of the heart in conversation with the deity. And yet, for all its simplicity, a profound depth is revealed in the human soul when it reaches beyond itself, indeed beyond the limits of its own world, and stretches out into the infinite mystery of God."[9]

Families in the autism community can give us encouragement as we are traveling down our path and experiencing God's grace and mercy. In the book of Hebrews, we are told to challenge and encourage each other toward love and doing the right thing, and to not give up on meeting with other believers, which we know all too well is easy to abandon (10:24–25).

After offering support to other autism parents at her son's school, one mother wrote, "There is peace in actually meeting a person who has made it through the worst autism has to offer and knowing there is light at the end of the tunnel. The power of peer support removes the isolation and allows us to move forward."[10]

Families with children who have autism may feel rejected by their relatives, society, or even the church, but an autism network can provide acceptance. In fact, disabled adults and parents of neurodivergent children tend to stay away from church for fear of not being accepted. What if my child has a meltdown and is seen as the naughty child? What if his behaviors scare other children? What if the volunteers for the special needs class don't show up today and my child disrupts the worship service? These are very real concerns for many people.

My best advice is to look until you find an autism-friendly church who loves your family unconditionally. Need a few ideas for where to start your search? You can start by asking other Christian friends with children on the spectrum where they attend church. Try googling churches in your area that advertise programs for those with special needs or sensory-sensitive services. Perhaps ask your current church if they have a buddy program, where a neurotypical person acts as a guide or works one-on-one with their child. And you can look for programs that may interest your child such as Bible memorization clubs or video game nights.

My friend Pastor Stephen J. Bedard, a father of five children, two of whom have autism, says: "Autistic children do weird things and make loud noises. Sort of like typical children, only better, and unfortunately more annoying to people who are not informed. You see, often there is no physical sign that an autistic child has anything wrong and when they act out, other adults glare at the parents for not keeping them under control. So for most parents, it is easier to just stay home from church. However, with the difficulties of raising a child with autism, a church community is exactly what a family needs."[11]

Friends stand by our side, quirks and all, and follow Scripture's command to demonstrate Christ's love and provide us with fellowship. Acts

2:46 says, "Every day they continued to meet together in the temple courts. They broke bread in their homes and ate together with glad and sincere hearts." And Proverbs 17:17 tells us, "A friend loves at all times, and a brother is born for a time of adversity."

> It's important to sometimes feel uncomfortable or like something is missing, because it's that feeling that forces us to go to God to find our ultimate comfort and community.

I am not trying to imply that community can solve all of our problems. Even in community and fellowship, we will still experience seasons of loneliness and worry. In some ways, it's important to sometimes feel uncomfortable or like something is missing, because it's that feeling that forces us to go to God to find our ultimate comfort and community.

My father-in-law, Bob, demonstrated the traits of a healing community by his love and acceptance of my autism.

My in-laws did not know I was diagnosed with autism when I married their daughter Kristen in 2012. They learned of my diagnosis in 2015 by my Facebook post announcing I received a contract for my book *A Parent's Guide to Autism*. My mother-in-law, after reading the post, called Kristen and exclaimed, "I didn't know Ron had autism! I just thought he was really eccentric and passionate about his interests."

After dating only a week, Kristen had invited me to her parents' house for a barbecue. My father-in-law, Bob, quickly realized I had some unusual quirks. As he placed the steaks on the grill, I jumped from my lawn chair, in the process spilling Mountain Dew on my shorts, and with hyper-speed I began to chase a gray baby bunny. Determined to escape my grasp, the bunny hopped under a pine tree. I was hot on her trail, crawling into the spiky terrain.

For the next hour, my future in-laws watched as I pursued a rabbit across the neighborhood, crawling under trees and into bushes. Finally, with steaks now cold as ice, I caught the gray-and-white fur ball.

Exhausted, I exclaimed, "I got the bunny! We can now eat." If that autistic episode wasn't enough to make my future in-laws realize I was on the spectrum, nothing would. Kristen fell in love with the rabbit and we named her Babs. Now Makayla enjoys chasing Babs around the apartment and seeing her hide under the couch.

After learning of my diagnosis, my father-in-law, an avid golfer, saw an ad for Ernie Els's The Els Center of Excellence in his favorite golfing magazine. "You need to contact The Els Center of Excellence and speak there," he told me. I contacted the director and was invited to be the keynote speaker of their first conference "Awe in Autism" in April of 2016.

Bob showed his love and acceptance of autism by driving me from their home in New Smyrna Beach to Jupiter, Florida, for the conference. This conference was the beginning of my autism speaking tours around the country. I currently serve as a young adult advisory board member for The Els Center of Excellence.

For our second anniversary, Kristen and I went with her parents to Israel. I loved seeing the Holy Land with the in-laws and even got to baptize my mother-in-law in the Jordan River. I loved climbing the 758-meter, truncated cone-shaped hill to the palace of Herod the Great. The wildlife on the hike was amazing—we saw Nubian ibex, a desert-dwelling goat species, and the rock hyrax, a small furry mammal. I quoted to my father-in-law, "Hyraxes are creatures of little power, yet they make their home in the crags" (Proverbs 30:26). Hyraxes also can spot danger from more than three thousand feet away. Bob and I shared a love of reading the Bible and historical facts.

After my father-in-law passed away, I received a ring he brought back from Jerusalem. It's a spinner ring; it's a typical band ring with an additional ring around it that spins freely. Engraved on the ring in Hebrew is the Shema, comprised of verses from both the biblical books of Numbers and Deuteronomy: "Hear, O Israel: The LORD our God, the LORD is one. Love the LORD your God with all your heart and with all your soul and with all your strength" (see Deuteronomy 6:4–5). I wear this ring to my speaking engagements and spin it when I get nervous. It reminds me to be the type of godly man Bob was, placing God first and making time for family and friends. Bob demonstrated his love and acceptance by always telling us, "If there is anything you need, just let me know." Our family misses Bob deeply, but I remember him as an example of what it means to be in community, and I try to extend that kindness to others around me.

CLOSING THOUGHTS

Whether our children are neurotypical or neurodivergent, life never turns out as expected or planned. In a broken world, nobody gets out unbroken, but a healing community can give us support in our battles, ideas for our frustrations, and power to help us grow closer to Christ. Rachel Marie Martin, an author and single mother of seven, says, "Sometimes you have to let go of the picture of what you thought life would be like and learn to find joy in the story you are actually living."[12]

PRAYER AND MEDITATION

Prayer

God, I have experienced deep sorrow—life has not turned out the way I expected. Please provide me with your comfort and peace. Bring people to encourage me with your Word and wisdom. Help me not to be isolated in my pain but to find healing through fellowship and community. When I am down, lift me up with your love and grace. Amen.

Meditation

All praise to God, the Father of our Lord Jesus Christ. God is our merciful Father and the source of all comfort. He comforts us in all our troubles so that we can comfort others. When they are troubled, we will be able to give them the same comfort God has given us. For the more we suffer for Christ, the more God will shower us with his comfort through Christ. (2 Corinthians 1:3–5 NLT)

Serve one another humbly in love. (Galatians 5:13)

PART 3

Thriving

Chapter 11

Learning to Communicate

*If I could snap my fingers and be nonautistic,
I would not. Autism is part of what I am.*

—Temple Grandin, *Thinking in Pictures*

*For you created my inmost being;
you knit me together in my mother's womb.*

—Psalm 139:13

Autism caused me to feel different as a child—like an endangered species. I remember in kindergarten attending a birthday party wearing a cowboy outfit, complete with boots and a ten-gallon hat. I loved the sensation of swinging the cowboy hat by its string. The problem was, I kept hitting other children in the face as I swung my hat. After this Wild West stimming incident, none of the other kids wanted to be my friend. I felt alone and isolated.

During the middle school years, bullying and a lack of friends made me question everything: Why did God make me like this? Why can't I control my feelings? What is my purpose in life?

Looking to the Bible helped me to deal with these natural questions.

In chapter 9 of John, when Jesus's disciples saw a man born blind, they inquired, "Rabbi, who sinned, this man or his parents, that he was born blind?" (verse 2). Jesus doesn't answer his disciples with the *cause* of disability. Instead, he answers by sharing the *purpose* of disability: It wasn't that anyone had done anything wrong. It was so that "the power of God could be seen" (verse 3 NLT).

Through my autism and other weaknesses, Christ displays his glory and strength. Second Corinthians 12:9 says, "'My grace is sufficient for you, for my power is made perfect in weakness.' Therefore I will boast all the more gladly about my weaknesses, so that Christ's power may rest on me."

Having autism is not easy, but God has given me special access to his power and grace because of my disabilities. This is especially true when I share my testimony in secular high schools and colleges. While most of those schools would never permit an average adult to share their faith, it's politically incorrect to tell an autistic adult not to speak about his special interest. Since my special interests are the Bible and Christ, public schools and colleges allow me to share my faith and its impact on my life. God uses my weakness of autism for me to be a missionary to the academic world.

> Communication and relationship skills—
> including friendship and career skills—are
> necessary to prepare young adults with autism for
> the most independent life they can possibly live.

That doesn't mean it's been an easy journey. In fact, I was not always a great communicator. Like Moses, I was slow in speech and went through difficult circumstances to learn how to be an effective communicator.

But communication and relationship skills—including friendship and career skills—are necessary to prepare young adults with autism for the most independent life they can possibly live. With those skills, a person with autism can live the life God created them to have with the purpose God wove into them.

Anita Lesko, a nurse anesthetist with autism, shares:

> The job market is highly competitive for everyone, even neuro-typicals. For those on the autism spectrum, it's far more difficult. But it's up to parents to get your kids out there doing various jobs at an early age. Start them at home doing chores. Something. Anything. Always, however, be sure of the child's safety.
>
> Having autism and working a career-type job is like going to a foreign country, not speaking their language, and trying to survive. To this day, all these years later, I still feel like a foreigner in a strange land. Yet I've built enough experience and "learned the language" enough to have a successful career. I know without a doubt in my mind that I would never have made it as an anesthetist if I hadn't had all my previous jobs.[1]

Only 5 percent of individuals with autism are gainfully employed. Thankfully, my dad was able to impart his work ethic—work hard, be disciplined, live frugally—to me.

When I was twelve years old, I was doing what I was able to do—cutting our acre lawn with a heavy push lawn mower for ten dollars a week. I had my first job outside the home at age fourteen as a busboy at Bill Knapp's. Having a job from an early age helped me learn life skills such as budgeting and saving money, dealing with angry customers, making friends with coworkers, and developing a healthy self-esteem.

It also prepared me for the next steps. Dr. Temple Grandin said, "Talent attracts mentors."[2] My junior year of high school, I began memorizing Scriptures (remember our discussion on harnessing special interests?). By the end of my senior year, I could quote over 2,000 verses. My Bible memory ability enabled me to be the first intern for international television evangelist Dr. Jack Van Impe, also known as "The Walking Bible." Dr. Van Impe taught me to memorize the Scriptures by subject on three-by-five-inch index cards, which I still keep in plastic boxes. I review each memory card every few weeks. I use my memory work as a coping skill to stay calm, feeling more connected to God through the Scriptures.

While good communication skills are essential for employment, it's also important for socialization. Even children who are nonverbal can develop some communication skills because not all communication is verbal: a hug expresses affection, a smile shows desire to socialize, and a frown conveys inward sorrow. For me, learning to express my emotions and interpret body language empowered me to control my feelings and develop friendships.

> Even children who are nonverbal can
> develop some communication skills because
> not all communication is verbal.

Despite my speech delays and difficulties with social interactions, my parents discovered three ways to help me learn to communicate and develop friendships.

1. All behavior is communication, so it's important to learn to decode your child's behavior and actions.

When a child is nonverbal or limited in speech, it's natural to have an outburst or meltdown when a need is not being met. Not being understood can be overwhelming and, as a result, an outburst or meltdown may be the child's only method for communication.

Carly Fleischmann, who is nonverbal but able to type, describes her struggles with sensory issues: "Autism feels hard. It's like being in a room with the stereo on full blast. It feels like my legs are on fire and over a million ants are climbing up my arms. It's hard to be autistic because no one understands me. People just look at me and assume that I am dumb because I can't talk or because I act differently than them. I think people get scared with things that look or seem different than them."[3]

My mom studied my behavior to understand my communication. When I was tapping my finger to my forehead or pacing in circles, this meant I was anxious or receiving too much stimulation. When I carried a small stuffed animal around the house, it meant I was feeling calm and wanted my mom to read to me or draw pictures.

When my mom was confronted by my out-of-control meltdowns, she would remind herself, "I am the adult. Ronnie needs me to stay calm and figure out what his problem is." When my daughter, Makayla, was young, she was typically a compliant child, unless she was hungry. I'm pretty sure she's the reason the term *hangry* was invented.

Keeping a journal of behavior and observations is a great way to help decipher what your child is trying to communicate.

Once you understand what needs and wants your child is communicating, you can begin to help them learn more socially acceptable ways of communicating those needs. In Makayla's case, when she was very young and "hangry," we would say, "I'm hungry. Food, please," then give her some food. As she matured, she was able to make the connection between her hunger and the need for food, then ask in an acceptable way.

2. Communication thrives with social interaction at home and in the community.

One of the best ways to help improve your child's social skills is providing consistent exposure to normal activities. Community events like activities at your local library or church youth group are a way to help your child interact in a social setting. With a bit of education for the leadership, these places and activities can be not only "safe" places for you and your child, but also an environment to help your child learn and thrive.

But you don't have to go outside your home to teach your child communication skills. Your child can also learn to communicate with simple things like household chores, because they require negotiation and problem-solving skills.

Parenting expert Katherine Reynolds Lewis shares the importance of family chores: "Adults think they're helping children by doing these tasks themselves, or outsourcing them. In fact, not giving them simple household chores deprives kids of the chance to build skills and be useful. Just think about how disorienting and demoralizing it is for adults to find themselves jobless—is it any surprise that children without any real responsibilities are increasingly anxious and depressed? Moreover, parents miss the opportunity to connect with kids while teaching them cleaning, laundry, cooking, bike repair, lawn work, and other necessary tasks."[4]

Of course the chores need to be appropriate for the skill level of your child. But children with autism love routines, and family chores can be a daily routine. Have your child do his chores at the same time each day, after dinner, or before homework. This will teach him to be organized, boosting self-confidence as well as raising his sense of responsibility. There are any number of family chores that children of all ages and abilities can accomplish: loading or unloading the dishwasher, setting the table for a meal, learning to cook, folding or putting away clothes, washing their own laundry, tidying their room each day, feeding or walking pets. In fact, a meaningful job could be as simple as turning on certain outdoor security lights when it gets dark out each night.

3. Friendships develop through communication.

Teach your child to be an active listener and ask for clarification to avoid misunderstandings. Active listening requires your child to ask relevant questions of the speaker, not to interrupt in the conversation, and also to repeat back what they hear. A fun activity you can do to sharpen active listening skills is read stories to your child and ask them to predict what will happen next. The prediction requires your child to listen to the details to make a logical guess.

The toughest part of communication for me was to think before I spoke and not bore people by my ramblings related to special interests. I have learned to pause before I speak—not saying the first thing that comes to mind—and then, when I do speak, I am brief, yet specific. Proverbs 17:28 says, "Even fools are thought wise if they keep silent, and discerning if they hold their tongues." I have learned the hard way that people don't want to be friends with a know-it-all; they desire friends who are interested in the things that interest them and who provide a listening ear.

Chase Sibary: Learning to Communicate Through Patience and Resilience

Bina Sibary quickly noticed a difference between her son Chase and his two older siblings.[5] Around five months, Bina realized Chase was not bonding with her like he should. He wasn't mimicking, babbling, cooing, or reacting to sounds and expressions.

Chase was an early walker and was getting on his feet around nine to ten months old. Around this time, he started to show some patterned behaviors and wouldn't respond to his name. Brian and his wife, Bina, thought Chase might have hearing problems and had him tested. To their surprise, the test revealed Chase could hear sounds they couldn't.

During Chase's first-year appointment, Brian and Bina shared their concerns with the pediatrician, and he provided them with a twenty-five-question test. Fearing the outcome, they answered no to seven questions when they should have answered yes. Holding back this information delayed the diagnosis. Chase began to miss milestones for speech. He wouldn't use any form of effective communication and later was diagnosed with apraxia, a motor disorder caused by damage to the brain in which the individual has difficulty with the motor planning to perform tasks or movements.

Chase did learn to communicate by pointing at objects and using the Picture Exchange Communication System, which allowed him to communicate using pictures. He showed signs of sensory processing disorder early and was hyposensitive to touch. He was very orally defensive to food, with different textures making him regurgitate. At an early age, Chase jumped off objects and landed hard, as well as ran into walls with his hands to define his surroundings.

At Chase's sixteen-month appointment, the Sibarys took another test; this time they answered yes to every question. The pediatrician had them schedule an evaluation with the local school district. After the evaluation, the educational specialists shared their concerns with Chase's development and suggested they set up an appointment with a neurologist for an official diagnosis. Chase was diagnosed with autism at two and a half years old.

Brian shares, "My wife and I handled the diagnosis differently. Bina was absolutely devastated and numb after seeing his low scores and the evaluation results. She started to grieve the life she wanted for Chase and our family. She was nervous about his future. At the same time, her motherly instincts kicked in and she began to aggressively research services for him. Bina's diligence and recognizing the early signs resulted in Chase quickly receiving early intervention and therapy.

"I felt sad for my son and knew I needed to learn about his diagnosis and how I could help him. I was determined to keep a positive attitude and decided to enjoy each moment and be thankful for such a beautiful boy. Our goal was for Chase to live the best life he can. To accomplish this we researched and did everything we could to get him in front of the right people at the right time that could help him in areas he struggled."

The greatest challenge for Brian and Bina was adjusting their family's life around therapy visits and travel to therapy locations, along with having two other children, ten years apart, who were living completely different lives.

"We don't shy away from doing whatever it takes to help Chase, but our lives revolved around long days," Brian explains. "Chase had therapy at Oakland University in Rochester, Michigan. His therapy there lasted for four hours, so my wife would stay onsite. This prevented her from working and tightened our budget so we could pay for therapy. After he was done with therapy at Oakland, he began at the Kaufman Center in West Bloomfield. Chase and Bina started the day leaving for therapy around 7:30 a.m. to be at the Kaufman Center by 9:00 a.m. He was picked up at 4:00 p.m. and arrived home around 5:30 p.m. This started when Chase was four and a half and lasted until he was seven and a half. Chase stopped attending the Kaufman Center at the end of May 2019.

"Our oldest son plays baseball and participated in many school functions. Throughout his high school career, baseball and other school events could only be attended by one parent. The other parent was with Chase. We couldn't afford to pay for a babysitter. Chase likes to explore, and getting him to sit still at an event is impossible. My wife and I have always said we feel like divorced parents since we are rarely together enjoying events as a family."

After years of only minimal progress, the Sibary family's hope was finally refreshed when Chase began learning sign language at the Kaufman Center. Bina shares, "We were shocked at how quickly Chase began to learn and use sign to communicate. At the same time, the therapist at the Kaufman Center started to address his apraxia. Within a short period of time, he was starting to sound out letters. This is when we started to gain hope he could communicate and possibly begin to talk.

"I don't know if there was ever a breakthrough moment, but there was a breakthrough year. Slow growth between the ages of five and six with language started to open up a whole new world for Chase and our family."

Each therapy Chase had received over the years prepared him for the next. When he arrived at the Kaufman Center for his apraxia treatment with speech therapy, all the prior ABA therapy at OU prepared him to be able to sit at a table during therapy. He understood how to sit in place, take direction, mimic, and how to work for a therapist. He was beginning to learn how others communicated with him.

Speech therapy instructed Chase to correctly position his mouth, tongue, and jaw to begin pronouncing letter sounds. Letters turned into small chunks of words, small chunks of words turned into full words, and full words turned into sentences so he could communicate with his parents and therapists.

Occupational therapy helped Chase with his sensory processing disorder. Now, he is able to tolerate more stimulation than he was able to in the past. Chase still seeks pressure, but not as often as he used to, and he has become more tolerant to sounds within his environment. His therapists have also worked on his strength and textures, and his vestibular, fine motor, and handwriting skills.

Throughout all of this, Brian's and Bina's faith in Christ provided them with hope. Brian says, "We know God is always watching over us and Chase. During seasons of distress, we can lean on him in prayer."

The Sibarys take particular comfort in Isaiah 41:10: "So do not fear, for I am with you; do not be dismayed, for I am your God. I will strengthen you and help you; I will uphold you with my righteous right hand." They also find strength in Joshua 1:9: "Be strong and courageous! Do not be afraid or discouraged. For the LORD your God is with you wherever you go" (NLT).

Chase has many passions in life and loves to be around water. Brian shares, "We have season passes at Cedar Point and Michigan's Adventure for the waterparks and slides. Chase enjoys the waves at Lake Michigan and playing in the sand at the beaches or in his sandbox. He also likes to ride his bike. He loves to explore new areas and map them out in his mind. Our bike rides usually range from eight to ten miles long."

Bina adds, "Chase likes to jump on trampolines, play at bounce houses, and music. The last two summers, Chase worked with music teachers, learning new songs. He loves to put together puzzles. Some days he will go through ten to fifteen different puzzles and quickly identify the location of the pieces. Exploring new apps on his iPad and seeing how they work is his current hobby."

Chase has taught Brian and Bina valuable lessons. As Bina explains, they now have "patience, resilience, and hope. Chase works really hard and enjoys the work. He has never resisted therapy and now that his therapy has been dialed back, he is asking to attend more. He misses his special friends, the therapists he developed relationships with. Chase overcame some big hurdles with his apraxia and sensory processing disorder. Through his hard work and determination, now at the age of eight, he is doing things we never thought he would."

Brian and Bina's advice to parents is, "Never give up hope and always stay positive. Try to stay away from negative thinking. Focus on providing the best support you can for your child with autism. Allow expectations to disappear and give your child the chance to amaze you with little milestones. Find support wherever you can. It may be from support groups, conferences, other families who have children with autism, or family and friends. When all the chips seem to be down, pray for strength and support."

CLOSING THOUGHTS

God has created your child in his image to display his glory. Your child is handmade by the Father with a purpose only he or she can accomplish. Learn to decode your child's behavior and actions. Encourage your child to interact socially with family chores, volunteer work, and involvement in the community. Communication empowers your child for friendships, independence, and employment.

PRAYER AND MEDITATION

Prayer

God, you created my child in your glorious image with a plan and purpose. You know my child completely. Father, reveal to me by your Holy Spirit ways to teach my child to communicate and interact socially. Teach me to focus on my child's abilities and stay positive. Amen.

Meditation

> Your eyes saw my unformed body; all the days ordained for me were written in your book before one of them came to be. (Psalm 139:16)

> Being confident of this, that he who began a good work in you will carry it on to completion until the day of Christ Jesus. (Philippians 1:6)

Chapter 12

Capturing the Moment

At the end of the day, the most overwhelming key to a child's
success is the positive involvement of parents.

—JANE D. HULL, GOVERNOR OF ARIZONA (1997–2003)

And so, dear brothers and sisters, I plead with you to give your
bodies to God because of all he has done for you. Let them be a
living and holy sacrifice—the kind he will find acceptable.
This is truly the way to worship him.

—ROMANS 12:1 (NLT)

BONDING WITH PEOPLE on the spectrum is difficult. But it is possible for
your family to be a cohesive unit if you learn to capture the moments in
front of you. Some of the rewards of being involved in your children's
lives are lasting memories, conversations, connectedness, and the chance
to watch your children grow into healthy, responsible adults. It can be a
challenge to make time for your children, but the more involved you are,
the more valued they will feel, and the more likely they will be to respond
to you.

I have discovered five ways for parents to have a positive involvement in their children's lives, both from how my parents raised me and from my own experience raising my daughter, Makayla.

1. Read Scriptures and pray at bedtime.

Every night, my parents would spend time reading the Bible and praying. We prayed for God's provision and guidance and for friends and relatives who were sick or in need of a miracle. It shows that you trust God and gives an example for your children to follow.

My dad wasn't a seminarian or pastor, but his simple reading of the Scriptures and praying formed the foundation for my brother and me that inspired us both to become ministers.

2. Give undivided attention to your children.

When I am on my computer writing my books, autism causes me to be self-absorbed and oblivious to my surroundings. Four-year-old Makayla demands, "Daddy, off computer. Chase me." Makayla loves for me to race with her around the house, jump on our bed, or sing and dance to the Mickey Mouse Club House "Hot Dog" song. I often have the song stuck in my head the next day at work, but it's worth it to see my daughter laughing and enjoying time with me.

> Giving attention to your children
> requires you to invest time doing
> activities they love to do.

As a kid, I loved when my dad played catch with me in the front yard. Make both dinnertime and bedtime free from electronic devices—for your kids *and* you. Being purposeful in not looking at a phone while your child is talking sets a good example for them to follow. Giving attention to your children requires you to invest time doing activities they love to do—it's never wasted time because it helps you to bond and grow closer as a family. If we spend time with our kids now, they are more likely to spend time with us later.

3. Take family vacations.

A study by the University of Toronto revealed parents are better off spending their money on vacations than on toys. The emotional response of any person when they have a cool experience creates an emotional connection that an object, such as a toy, simply cannot. And there are so many types of experiences to choose from: close to home or far away; calming or heart pumping; full of relaxation or full of activity; inexpensive or extravagant.

Since I loved prairie dogs and wildlife, my favorite family vacation was when we went for two months out west and saw moose, elk, pika, wolves, and grizzly bears at Yellowstone National Park. "An 'enriched' environment offers new experiences that are strong in combined social, physical, cognitive, and sensory interaction," says child psychotherapist Dr. Margot Sunderland.[1] All of these interactions are particularly important for kids on the spectrum.

> Because a person with autism has a differently wired brain, making the effort to join your child in "their" world will give you glimpses of the world—their world— from an entirely different point of view.

Family vacations provide your child with lasting memories, social interaction, and educational experiences. Vacations don't have to break the bank; you can camp locally or at a state park for a price within your budget. Children with autism love traditions since they follow routines. One tradition my family followed was having sugar cereal like Boo Berry on Saturday mornings and on vacations. On family vacations my parents would get each of us a souvenir. Another friend involved their autistic child in planning the structure for the day and the order of events that would happen each day of vacation.

Just a reminder: be careful not to define vacation in a super traditional way. Your child is not traditional—and neither is your family—and a visit to Yellowstone National Park might not be a good fit for your family.

Sometimes a day trip to a favorite park and restaurant can provide the precious memories and bonding you all desire.

4. Eat dinners together.

During dinner, my parents would have each family member share what happened during their day. My dad told humorous stories about his coworkers at General Motors, and I would talk about track and cross-country practice. Eating my mom's spaghetti and meatballs with a large glass of milk made this experience even more enjoyable!

Dr. Anne Fishel, one of the founders of The Dinner Project, shares amazing findings about family dinners. "Most of us know intuitively that family dinners are good for families. Dramatic research findings show that family dinners can also inoculate us against a host of ills, from substance abuse and obesity to low achievement scores and behavioral problems. Studies show that dinner conversation is an even more potent vocabulary-booster for our children than reading to them. Other studies show that the stories that we tell around the kitchen table help our children to build resilience and self-esteem."[2] Ultimately, eating family meals creates a strong unity in the family to help overcome adversity.

5. Enter your child's world by taking an interest.

Because a person with autism has a differently wired brain, making the effort to join your child in "their" world will give you glimpses of the world—their world—from an entirely different point of view.

Pastor Jason Hague's son, Jack, is functionally nonverbal. He shares that the best way he is able to enter Jack's world is "through his movies. Jack loves Pixar and DreamWorks films, and he can quote them. We all became experts in his movies. We know the lines, we know the songs. My sons will act out entire scenes from movies like *Up* or *Ratatouille*.

"My daughters will paint pictures or make clay characters from *Kung Fu Panda* or *Monsters, Inc.* And I will talk to him in the voices of Gru, Mike Wazowski, or Lightning McQueen. I especially love to use the voices of the father characters from those movies, because that really resonates with him. When we've become more intentional about stuff like this, he has opened up more and more.

"Some of Jack's world is colorful and fun and hilarious. One day, he was sitting on the back of our car and fell off in the driveway. His big sister ran to him and said, 'Jack, are you okay?' and the situation must have reminded him of a scene in *Kung Fu Panda* when Po, the panda, rushes in to see if Master Shifu is still alive. Jack looked at his sister and stole Shifu's line: 'I'm not dead, you idiot!' She about fell down laughing. I love seeing those glimpses into his world, and I love it when he shows us something new."[3]

When I need advice or prayer, I call my parents. I am still close to my parents because they both invested quality time in my life and created lasting memories. They have encouraged me not to be so busy with work and presenting that I neglect the thing that matters most: family.

As we bond and connect with our children we create lasting memories and empower our sons and daughters to transition into adulthood.

Malcolm Wang: Using Photography for Connection and Bonding

On March 9, 2018, I met Malcolm Wang, a sixteen-year-old photographer and autism self-advocate and his mom, Karen, at the Autism Alliance of Michigan's fourth annual Navigating Autism conference.[4] I was presenting a breakout session on *Autism, Athletics, and Activities* and my book table was next to Malcolm's photograph exhibit.

We talked about autism and advocacy and quickly became friends. Malcolm shared how he developed social skills by participating in autism conferences and photography exhibits. "I learned to talk more with people. People are nice once you start talking to them."

Communication and social interaction did not come naturally for Malcolm as a child due to sensory issues. "I was sensitive to noise. Loud sounds hurt my ears. I was sensitive to food and texture. I am sensitive to feeling air on my skin. I always wear long sleeves, even in the summer. I am sensitive to bright sunlight, but transition lenses help with that. I had trouble falling asleep. I woke up during the night and my mom would have to stay with me."

His mother, Karen, shares, "Malcolm was diagnosed with autism spectrum disorder when he was three years old because of his panic attacks;

it was not possible to get a clear evaluation before then because he would have a panic attack at any building that resembled a doctor's office and elope before the evaluation. We knew his development was not following a typical pattern, but we were repeatedly told by family, friends, and physicians that we were just nervous, first-time parents, and things would get better if we calmed down. So we always knew he was different, but we couldn't explain exactly what was going on. It was very confusing, and the lack of understanding was devastating for us. My faith is what pulled me through that period."

While on vacation, Malcolm's parents noticed his incredible memory ability and love of numbers. This love of numbers would later inspire his photography artwork. When he was two years old, the family went to visit his grandpa in Wisconsin and stayed in hotel room 413. A year and a half later, his family stayed in the same hotel. While his parents were checking in at the front desk, Malcolm went to room 413. Amazed, Malcolm's parents had to explain to their three-year-old they were staying in 409 this time.

Now, Malcolm's love for numbers is seen in his photos. "I love taking pictures of trail markers at state parks and nature preserves. The trail markers are special because they are numbered and they have a picture of the park map. I love to memorize the maps and the numbers. From taking pictures of trail markers, I learned to focus the camera. I look at the trail marker pictures at home on the computer and it makes me feel happy and brings back a happy memory."

Malcolm still enjoys memorizing parking spots and hotel room numbers. In Detroit, he and his Uncle Mike parked in spot 4101 for a baseball game. Three times, Malcolm questioned his uncle, "What spot are we in?" to test his memory.

Feigning ignorance, his Uncle Mike would continually ask, "Where are we parked?"

This become an inside joke between them—now Uncle Mike and Malcolm text each other back and forth about spot 4101.

Malcolm's parents connected with him by family vacations, numbers, and photography. But the connecting didn't simply end there.

Malcolm's second love is nature, cultivated by his mom. "She took me for long walks every single day. We went in the woods and around the block. She took me to see things that were interesting to me like fountains and tall buildings. If I woke up at 5 a.m. and could not go back to sleep, we would walk in the neighborhood or go to the twenty-four-hour grocery store or swimming at the recreation center. I learned the words for different things and about different places on our journeys. This satisfied my curiosity."

Malcolm's greatest challenge with autism was learning. "I had my first IEP when I was one and a half years old. I started speech therapy and occupational therapy. But I had so much anxiety and panic attacks that it was very hard for me to learn. For a long time, I had to practice being near noise, light, and people, and it took a long time for me to learn how to eat different types of food. The important thing is that I was able to learn. When I had the right kind of help, I could do things just like other kids."

In elementary and middle school, Malcolm attended cross-categorical classrooms and general education classrooms. He had difficulty developing friendships and understanding the lessons. Malcolm's family moved to Northville, Michigan, after fourth grade for a better learning environment. It was a good choice. Northville teachers helped him with reading comprehension and math. He took social skills classes at school and at the Friendship Circle. On Sundays, Malcolm attended Sunday school and was an altar boy.

Through the spiritual disciplines and church, Malcolm learned to handle his panic attacks. "Praying and going to church keeps me calm when I feel anxious. When I was having panic attacks every day, I would ask mom to take me to church. When I walked into the quiet church, I calmed down. I felt love and peace inside. I love hearing the holy gospel at church. I also love receiving Holy Communion at church. At the church I attended, Sacred Heart Byzantine Catholic Church, everything is chanted. Most of the prayers are repeated. So it's easy to learn. When things are repeated and chanted, it makes me feel calm and happy. It's easy to understand."

Malcolm advocates for inclusion in religious services. "When I am not serving, I sit in the front row. I can see everything and participate in the liturgy with all the prayers and songs. When there is a fundraiser at church, I volunteer. I set up for the church garage sale and help with the coatroom at the ladies' tea. I think some churches are afraid of autistic behaviors. They should not be afraid. They should include everyone. They should let people participate using their gifts for God's glory." In sixth grade, Malcolm's passion for photography was born. "I liked to press buttons on cameras. I liked to look at pictures. As a child, I loved to press elevator buttons, and when I did chores, I enjoyed pressing the dishwasher and washing machine buttons. I also liked to flip light switches on and off. My parents encouraged my interest in photography by having me take pictures of my family members."

Malcolm, through photography, captures the beauty of nature. "I started taking pictures of nature in 2013 when I was twelve years old. I saw trees, birds, flowers, and ponds. Every year in June, we go to the Nichols Arboretum in Ann Arbor to see the peonies in full bloom between trail markers one and two. Then, after we see the peonies and take lots of good pictures, we go see the other trail markers.

"My high school classes helped me enjoy photography even more. I took two semesters of photography, and I took a class in environmental science where I had to learn the names of animals and trees. Now, I find the animals and trees in the parks, and I name my photos after each species. In English class, I learned about figurative language like metaphors. So, my photography is a metaphor for my autistic worldview."

Malcolm captures the moment by spending time in nature. He goes on hiking adventures with his family to find the perfect pictures. "My favorite places to go hiking are state parks and botanical gardens. Last summer, I went to Michigan State University to participate in a research study, and I took photos of the flowers at the botanical gardens there."

The two types of cameras Malcolm uses reflect his artistic style. "The first is a small autofocus Canon PowerShot Elph 135 that I use to shoot photos through a kaleidoscope. Those are abstract photos with a repetitive pattern. I love my kaleidoscope photos because the pattern is different every time. I have thirteen kaleidoscope photos in my portfolio right now, but I am working on more. My other camera is a Canon PowerShot SX530 HS, and this is a digital SLR camera. I use that one for zooming in on flowers and insects. These photos have a higher resolution."

Music also empowered Malcolm to capture the moment. "People connect with music. When I was little it was very hard for me to understand words. My parents sang songs to help me understand the meaning of words and to help me calm down. My parents made up songs to teach me about everyday things like taking a bath, putting on socks, or going to school. These songs helped me learn about the world—things I could not understand by spoken language alone. Today I still love music. I am the official DJ of my family."

Malcolm received the Award of Excellence from the National Parent Teacher Association in the Reflections Art Competition in the Special Artist Category in 2016 for his photography. In 2017 and 2018, he won the Michigan PTA's Award of Excellence for his service in the community.

"My life today is very different from when I was a little boy. I still love books, and I still feel anxious sometimes. But, I understand more. I can tell people what I'm thinking and feeling. I can share my interests with other people. My specialty is nature photography. I do close-ups of trees, flowers, birds, and water. God created everything. When I take pictures of nature, I am taking pictures of creation. I consider myself a working artist. I sell prints and cards at local art fairs. I submit my photos to professional exhibits. I feel close to God and love in my heart all the time.

"One of my photos was displayed at the Matthaei Botanical Garden at the University of Michigan. It's a photo of flowers that I shot through a kaleidoscope. In 2017, I had my first solo exhibit at the Novi Civic Center's public gallery. I showed thirty-one photos in honor of autism awareness month. The exhibit was so successful, they invited me back to exhibit in 2018. I share the story of my photography because it shows how a special interest can develop and connect people together."

Malcolm graduated from high school in 2019 and is attending Michigan Career and Technical Institute. His current goals include participating with friends on fun road trips, continuing with photography and art shows, opening an Etsy shop, getting a job using his gifts, and, most importantly, bringing happiness to people and serving God, all while capturing moments with his gift of photography.

Malcolm's passion for art, music, and photography enables him to connect and bond with others—enjoying social activities with his friends like roads trips and photography shows.

CLOSING THOUGHTS

Positive involvement in your child's life creates memories and emotional connection. You can bond with your child by giving attention to his or her special interests and spending quality time together. These interests, like Malcolm's, can help your child learn social skills, experience life, enjoy nature, and grow spiritually.

PRAYER AND MEDITATION

Prayer

God, please help me to connect with my children, setting aside time to take an interest in the things that interest them. Show me fun activities to participate in with my family, and provide reminders that even simple things, like eating meals together, are healthy for every member of our family. Thank you for the promise that your Word is light to the path you have set our family on. I place my trust in you; direct my steps. Amen.

Meditation

Children are a gift from the LORD; they are a reward from him. (Psalm 127:3 NLT)

Let the children come to me. Don't stop them! For the Kingdom of Heaven belongs to those who are like these children. (Matthew 19:14 NLT)

Chapter 13

Living the Dream

Behold the turtle! He makes progress
only when his neck is out.
—James Bryant Conant, *Harvard to Hiroshima*

Why do you spend money for what is not bread, and your wages
for what does not satisfy? Listen carefully to Me, and eat what is
good, and let your soul delight itself in abundance.
—Isaiah 55:2 (NKJV)

Living the dream means living the life you want, without regret, while enjoying the fruits of your labor. For me, living the dream is enjoying time with my family, writing, and traveling the country speaking on autism and faith. Living the dream can mean different things to different people. Your dreams will change as your life circumstances change. As a child, I dreamed of playing professional baseball for the Oakland A's. As an adult, my dream career is using my gifts to help families with special needs children.

Even while living your dream, you'll experience struggles and moments of despair. This past year, we decided to adopt a puppy for our daughter, Makayla, despite living in a compact apartment with an aggressive calico cat named Frishma and a nocturnal dwarf rabbit named Babs. The first night with Rudy (a Jack Russell Terrier and Pomeranian mix with healthy vocal cords) was a nightmare.

The sleepless night began with our shy pup exploring his new home; then he got a scent of Babs, and his ears and tail shot up, his back muscles tightened, white fangs emerged, and he began snarling and barking with a sound that can best be described as a blood-curdling scream.

The rest of the night Rudy continually scratched at our bedroom door while whimpering with a high-pitched groan. In the background, we could hear Babs thumping her hind feet while banging the bars of her cage, and the sound of Frishma hissing and yowling.

We tried having Rudy sleep in his crate, only to discover we adopted a Houdini escape artist. The only thought that went through my mind was, "What did I just get myself into?" Rudy was finally able to relax and fall asleep in our bed at 2:30 a.m.

I don't know about you, but that sounds a bit like a metaphor for life with a child on the spectrum. You introduce one new element to the mix, and your world goes haywire. You are living the dream, then your child is diagnosed with autism and you're left trying to juggle therapy appointments, a job, other kids, and then look, the furnace dies and you're left shivering in a freezing cold house.

The good news is that our pet debacle didn't continue for long. A few days after introducing Rudy, we were enjoying the dream: Rudy and Frishma sitting next to each other on the couch, no longer arch nemeses; Babs calm in her cage eating her carrots.

Two-year-old Rudy now sleeps a full eight hours a night. And as I write, Rudy is living the dream too—sunbathing against the sliding glass door with no cares in the world.

And the fact is, no matter the challenges you face, you can still find joy and live the dream too.

Italians call this *bella vita*—beautiful life. It's a mindset, an attitude, and a lifestyle, an enthusiastic desire to live life to the fullest because the simple act of being alive is joyful itself.

As Ecclesiastes 2:24–25 says, "Nothing is better for a man than that he should eat and drink, and that his soul should enjoy good in his labor. This also, I saw, was from the hand of God. For who can eat, or who can have enjoyment, more than I?" (NKJV). Discover joy in your labor. I have fun taking Rudy outside for his restroom breaks. I put on my sweatpants and hit the trails for a short run. This helps me lose extra weight and reminisce about my glory days of cross-country while the run burns up a little bit of Rudy's endless supply of energy. For you, enjoying life might be reading an interesting book while waiting for your child to finish therapy or planning a family fun day.

> Striving for excellence instead of
> perfection frees me from anxiety.

Rabbi Marc Gellman encourages parents to strive for true happiness for their children and themselves. Gellman makes it clear that he's not simply talking about instant pleasure—the kind we get from a yummy bowl of ice cream, the type of happiness many people seek—but the true happiness that comes from doing hard but good things repeatedly—such as learning to enjoy celery or other healthful foods—and doing those things most of the time. A steady habit of instant pleasure leads to an unhealthy person; the other leads to really living life.[1]

I recommend five ways to live life with true happiness in the midst of chaos.

1. Let go of your perfectionist mindset.

Dr. Steve Greene writes, "[People] who seek perfection are rarely satisfied, often disappointed, and generally less productive. Perfectionists simply do not get as much done as [individuals] who accept excellence as their goal."[2] Perfectionism destroys our self-esteem with unrealistic expectations.

Striving for excellence instead of perfection frees me from anxiety. Learning from my mistakes and sharing my imperfections help me to be a better employee, husband, and dad.

If your child's occupational therapist has requested you to work with your child every day on a skill, but your week blew up, your child's exhausted, and you can only get five sessions in, it might be okay for that week.

Or perhaps you've been working on mitigating circumstances so your child doesn't melt down at the hair salon . . . and your child melts down again. Remind yourself that you're working toward improvement, and celebrate that you and your child were able to lessen the length and severity of the meltdown. And maybe this time you didn't melt down along with your child.

It hasn't always been easy, but at least my imperfections also provide humorous stories for my books.

2. Talk with your children about their emotions and honor them.

All children, whether neurotypical or neurodivergent, have difficulty processing negative emotions. As children encounter fear, sadness, anxiety, anger, and other negative emotions, parents need to help children identify and put words to those feelings. This is a step toward helping children along their journey of dealing with negative emotions in positive ways.[3]

Now, let's focus on neurodivergent children. Children with autism experience more difficulty monitoring and altering their emotions, since their emotional arousal is more like an on/off switch than a dial that increases and decreases gradually.

You can teach your children to control their emotions and maintain a calm state by focusing on solutions to the things that make them frustrated and encouraging them to verbalize their feelings or to take a time-out.

So perhaps before you have a difficult discussion with a child or take them to do something they hate, tell them what you're going to do, what your expectations are, and what the good and bad consequences will be. It allows your child to make a decision *before* they're in crisis mode. I have a friend who, when she has something difficult to discuss with her child with Asperger's, says, "I need to talk to you about something, but you might not like it. In fact, you might want to throw yourself on the ground and have a fit about it. So why don't you do that now so we can get it over with?" This usually earns her a grin and miraculously prevents a meltdown.

Just a word of warning that each child is at a different stage and should have varying standards. As we discussed in the last point, you'll be setting yourself and your child up for failure if you expect perfection, especially the first time around or for any length of time.

Dr. Stella Acquarone, a child psychologist and founder of Parent Infant Centre, says, "To be autistic means to be hypersensitive to emotions and other experiences. I always think that a baby or child with autistic behaviours is frightened, overwhelmed. They can't cope. It is important to reach those emotions that are so strong in them—fear, rage—and give them a way to express themselves, even if it's through drawing or song."[4] The more you can help your children develop a rich emotional vocabulary, the better prepared they'll be for the storms of adolescence and early adulthood.

3. Consider getting a pet to provide your child companionship and purpose.

Before you panic, hear me out. Many families with children on the spectrum feel like they are trapped at home due to their child's anxiety and meltdowns. But a therapy or comfort animal can help ease the transition for your child, creating a sort of link between home and other places.

One mom shares the story of how her son on the spectrum became so depressed that he wanted to simply disappear. Nothing seemed to help . . . until the day his mom brought home a therapy dog. This unconditional friendship was both life-changing and life-giving for her child. Leaving the house was, and still is, an anxiety-inducing exercise for the ten-year-old, but if his therapy dog accompanies him, his anxiety disappears and the entire process goes more smoothly.

Madden Humphreys, a seven-year-old from Oklahoma, has a rare eye condition, Heterochromia iridum, which causes his eyes to be two different colors: one hazel and the other blue. He also has a bilateral cleft lip. A member of an online cleft support group posted a rescue cat from the streets of Minnesota who had the same conditions as Madden. After seeing the cat's picture, Madden's mom, Christina, flew to Minnesota to adopt Moon.

In an interview with Kaitlyn Alanis of *The Wichita Eagle*, Christina shares, "We knew immediately that this kitty was meant to be part of our family. . . . We knew they were destined to be best friends." Having a pet with his same rare conditions helped Madden feel understood and less alone and to realize that being different doesn't make him a freak: it just makes him unique. Moon also caused Madden's self-esteem to soar.[5]

Anita Lesko, a nurse anesthetist and author of *Becoming an Autism Success Story*, shares her experience caring for horses and learning life skills: "The bottom line is that when I walked into that stable all those years ago, I felt trapped inside a shell, unable to join in life like everyone else. I was uncoordinated, timid, had zero self-esteem, and was unable to talk to anyone besides my mom. When I left to go to college, I was a different person: self-confident, coordinated, balanced. I had management skills, work skills, I knew how to interact with anyone, and I had discovered my ability to laser focus. Horses saved my life."[6]

The American Veterinary Medical Association affirms that there is a mutually beneficial relationship between humans and animals. This bond enhances the health and well-being of all involved parties.[7]

See, there was good reason for us to introduce Rudy the yipping pup into our home.

4. Be physically healthy to make life more enjoyable.

Physical health consists of nutrition and diet, exercise, controlling our stress and anxiety level, leisurely activities, medical care, and getting enough sleep and rest. Happiness researcher Dr. Robert Holden conducted a survey and found that 65 out of 100 people would choose happiness over health, but that both were highly valued.[8] Fortunately, we don't have to choose: happiness and health go together like peanut butter and jelly.

Think about it for a moment. If you have a fun day planned, but you're exhausted and hungry, you won't enjoy what otherwise would have been a fun day. Still don't believe me? Study after study shows that exercise both improves mood and boosts energy. Further, if we don't take care of our physical well-being, we cannot care for the needs of our children.

5. View life through a different lens.

Sometimes our dreams are the very things holding us back from finding joy. As hard as it is, we need to let go of the things we once expected and embrace the reality of where we are . . . then we can move forward into new hopes and dreams.

As you release the old and reassess what's truly possible, you might discover that that painful step now becomes your biggest leap into a future filled with true happiness.

Alix Generous: Confounding the Wise with a Beautiful Mind

The childhood of Alix Generous was clouded by misdiagnoses and dark depression.[9] As a baby, crowded malls caused her to cry hysterically. She was terrified by the sensation of bath water touching her fragile body and was extremely sensitive to certain textures of foods. For a three-month period of time, Alix chose to eat only tomato soup. She hated any clothing made of velvet. Just the thought of it would make her itch. Due to her hyperactive behavior and intense focus, psychiatrists misdiagnosed her as having attention deficit hyperactivity disorder.

When Alix was six years old, her severe depression and manic behavior caused her to receive a new misdiagnosis of bipolar disorder. At age eleven, a powerful antipsychotic medication caused Alix's jaw to lock, and medications to increase dopamine caused her to have hallucinations and other side effects. Alix shares, "The heavy medications I received as a child have caused me to have a difficult time recalling events of my life before age ten."

While Alix rode on the school bus in middle school, a young man bullied and sexually assaulted her. Shortly after, Alix's parents sent her for two years to a special treatment school in Provo, Utah. This school kept Alix on a strict schedule; when she refused to shower her first night there, the staff stayed up with her until she showered and then made her wake up at 6:45 a.m. After finishing the program in Utah, she attended

Olney Friends School, a Quaker boarding school in Ohio, from age fifteen until she graduated at seventeen.

Alix describes her depression: "When you are depressed, you don't feel things as they are—you have a block. Depression causes some people to want to stay in bed all day and accomplish nothing, but I made a conscious decision based on who I wanted to be rather than what I felt like. I decided to arise from my bed and fulfill my dreams. This act of choice over feelings and emotions enabled me to discover the world around me."

Alix was beginning to choose to enjoy life. As a child and young adult, Alix had a great love for music and animals. She could name every major musical from the late eighteenth century to the 1980s and taught herself to play the piano from hearing musicals. When she experienced anxiety and depression, music and riding horses helped her feel at peace. Alix currently relaxes by wearing her onesie and watching Netflix with her cat, Pooshka, and Chauncey, her autism service dog.

> "This world is in desperate need of creative and intellectual minds to solve complex problems. But before we can do that, we need to build a culture that accepts mental diversity."

The turning point in Alix's life occurred when she was twelve years old and was correctly diagnosed with Asperger's syndrome. "Life finally began to make sense, and I understood the way my brain processes information differently and the reason for my social awkwardness. My mind moves a thousand miles an hour. And in a split second, I'll have an idea that's three or four conversations ahead of where everyone else is, and I share it. I've been told that I use technical and, at times, overly formal vocabulary in everyday conversations. It's how my mind thinks."

As Raymond B. Fosdick, who served as president of the Rockefeller Foundation from 1936 to 1948, stated, "It is always the minorities that hold the key of progress; it is always those who are unafraid to be different that advance human society."[10] The apostle Paul said, "But God chose the foolish things of the world to shame the wise; God chose the weak things of the world to shame the strong" (1 Corinthians 1:27).

Through perseverance and dedication, Alix has learned to harness her beautiful mind, and at twenty-eight years old, she has accomplished more than many people do in a lifetime. "This world is in desperate need of creative and intellectual minds to solve complex problems. But before we can do that, we need to build a culture that accepts mental diversity." Alix has made a significant contribution to science, delivered a TED talk in June of 2015 that has received over two million views, and also delivered two other TED talks. When Alix was nineteen, she won a research competition for her scientific work in quorum sensing and coral reefs, which she presented to the United Nations in the fall of 2012. She was also one of the founders of the company, AutismSees (now called Podium for Autism), which provides online tools to equip individuals with autism to learn social skills and resources for employment.

When listening to Alix's most-viewed TED talk, I find it amazing to hear her graceful sense of humor. "You may have noticed that I don't have much inflection in my voice," she shares with the audience. "That's why people often confuse me with a GPS. This can make basic communication a challenge." She grins and says, "Unless you need directions."[11]

Alix encourages us to remember that "the world does not need more intelligent people; it just needs people who are kinder and willing to listen."

CLOSING THOUGHTS

Living the dream means to relax and not get caught up in life's rat race, allowing yourself to make mistakes without grieving, and living in the moment to enjoy both your family's and God's presence. In the book of Psalms, King David encourages his readers to *selah*: to pause to acknowledge the presence of God in creation. Psalm 46:10 says, "Be still, and know that I am God; I will be exalted among the nations, I will be exalted in the earth." As we are still before God and exalt him, we experience freedom from worry by acknowledging that God is bigger than our concerns.

Your dreams may be different now than when you first began parenting, and that's okay and it's common. With some changes in your expectations and with God's help, you can live in true happiness. You can live the dream.

PRAYER AND MEDITATION

Prayer

Refresh my heart, Father, helping me to relax and enjoy life. Fill me with the wonder of creation, the majesty of wildlife and nature: listening to the ducks quacking in the park, the birds chirping their songs. When I am anxious or afraid, be my protector and give me rest. Bless my journey with more laughter and joy. Children grow so quickly; let me not take one moment for granted. Amen.

Meditation

Are not two sparrows sold for a penny? Yet not one of them will fall to the ground outside your Father's care. And even the very hairs of your head are all numbered. So don't be afraid; you are worth more than many sparrows. (Matthew 10:29–31)

Come to me, all you who are weary and burdened, and I will give you rest. Take my yoke upon you and learn from me, for I am gentle and humble in heart, and you will find rest for your souls. For my yoke is easy and my burden is light. (Matthew 11:28–30)

Chapter 14

First Gleam of Dawn

An optimist is one who sees an opportunity in every difficulty.
A pessimist is one who sees a difficulty in every opportunity.
—L. P. JACKS

The path of the righteous is like the morning sun,
shining ever brighter till the full light of day.
—PROVERBS 4:18

THE FIRST GLEAM of dawn is the foretaste of the day's coming brightness. Early in the morning, while camping, I love to see the first gleam of dawn. This reminds me that a bright, sunny day awaits us, full of swimming, fishing, and hiking.

The best way to describe the first gleam of dawn is a scene from the movie *Pleasantville*. In the movie, a kid's whole world is black-and-white, until his town is suddenly transformed with color. The rising sun brings forth a new day and a fresh perspective on life.

After your child receives an autism diagnosis, things can seem dark and the outlook bleak, but don't stay stuck there. Watch for the glimmers of light that are coming. The first gleam of dawn is seeing that spark of hope which leads to development—maybe it's in speech or social interaction. Autism is characterized by developmental delays, but "delay" does not mean "never." It means you have to be patient and wait.

The first gleam of dawn occurred for world-class mile runner Mikey Brannigan, who was nonverbal until age five, as he was climbing on the jungle gym. Mikey was hanging on to the playground structure, looked straight at his mom, and said, "Help me!"

His mother, Edie, shares, "I fell to the ground, stunned, and began to cry because I knew that if he could communicate his needs, unprompted and with situational appropriateness, he could do anything."[1]

For my parents, the aha moment was Prairie Pup in 1982. The breakthrough moment for Brittany Tagliareni, whose story I share later in this chapter, was when she picked up a tennis racket at age sixteen.

When those first glimpses of dawn begin to peek through the clouds, we need to recognize and celebrate them, to celebrate our children. Here are four suggestions for what to do while waiting for those gleams of light and how to celebrate them when they do break through.

1. Don't let your child's limitations hold them or you back from enjoying life.

Most of the glimpses will be small. A fourteen-year-old boy asking for a hug at bedtime when he hasn't done that since he was two. A twelve-year-old girl looking her mom in the eye during a conversation without being reminded. For my mom the first glimpses were my learning to say the word *brother* and controlling my meltdowns in school.

> If you're waiting for your child to be perfect in every way, stop waiting, because it will never happen.

You can help your child move forward by encouraging him to participate in activities he enjoys. In eighth grade when Prairie Pup was expelled from school, my parents encouraged me to run on the track team. They bought me cool blue and neon-yellow Nike running shoes and attended all my track meets. I felt loved seeing my parents in the stands cheering for me.

If you're waiting for your child to be perfect in every way, stop waiting, because it will never happen. Every single person has imperfections and God still chooses to use us. The Bible talks about people God used in huge ways who had some pretty obvious limitations: Moses had a speech impediment (Exodus 4:10), the prophet Jeremiah had low self-esteem (Jeremiah 1:6–7), and the apostle Paul had a thorn in the flesh (2 Corinthians 12:7–9). God is the only perfect one.

CJ Hernandez was diagnosed with autism at the age of three. Due to sensory issues, he was terrified of haircuts. CJ shares, "What got me real intimidated was the clipper, how it makes the noise, and the shears. I thought they were going to cut my eyes out."[2] Now CJ has overcome his sensory issues and is employed as a barber at Jhonny's Barbershop in Avondale, Arizona. He's dubbed himself "The Autistic Barber" and styles the hair of children with autism who fear the barbershop. CJ displays his work on Instagram.

CJ had his own gleam of dawn when he overcame his fear of the barbershop and became a barber. Now he brings light to other children on the spectrum through his work.

2. Create a way to remember small breakthroughs.

Write small breakthrough moments in a journal, or create a visual remembrance. I have a portfolio reminding me of how far I have come. I have included pictures of my winning the Detroit Edison Poster Contest and mentoring under Dr. Jack Van Impe. I also have a section titled "Times of Testing" with IEP reports and evaluations from professionals describing how far behind my development was and how far I have come.

A cool example of a visual remembrance was a mom whose daughter had sensory issues and, after praying about it, accidentally discovered that turning the socks inside out made them tolerable. The mom now has her daughter's little sock pinned to a board in her room to remind her of the answered prayer.

3. Do something special to celebrate progress.

There are two sides of training your child—instruction and encouragement. Instruction consists of teaching your child appropriate behavior and how to interact socially. The encouragement is celebrating his progress and enjoying the journey.

When your child makes progress, take time to celebrate instead of moving straight on to the next life lesson they need to learn. Make a special dessert, do a movie night—whatever your family enjoys. My family celebrated my progress with blueberry frozen yogurt from the grocery store. When I was in high school my parents celebrated my academic success with a new Nintendo video game. My parents also celebrated by giving themselves a short, lakeside vacation.

When you celebrate your child's progress, you give him the courage to press forward and mature as he learns the lessons of life.

4. When facing delays and regression, never forget how far God has taken your family.

Raising a child on the spectrum can sometimes mean experiencing periods of regression, times of moving backward in the progress you've made.

One of my favorite family stories is about my grandparents' vacation to Florida. My grandpa began the twenty-four-hour drive in Michigan on I-75 south. Ten hours into the journey, he felt tired and had my grandma take the wheel. Rubbing his eyes as he woke from a deep sleep, he saw a sign: "Welcome to Michigan." My grandpa joked, "We finally got to sunny Florida—it just took us a little longer because my wife is directionally challenged."

New schools, peers, therapies, or teachers can lead to learning setbacks. When your child goes through a season of regression, watch for the gleams of dawn and, in the meantime, try to keep your sense of humor. As Grandpa said, "Sunny days are just around the corner . . . despite temporary delays."

Brittany Tagliareni: Giant Slayer

Thirty-year-old Brittany Tagliareni, at five feet, two inches tall and barely over a hundred pounds, is a little powerhouse on the tennis court.[3]

She has won more than one hundred medals and beat many of the top-ranked Special Olympics male athletes. Brittany's accomplishments have been featured on CNN, ESPN, and *The Today Show*. Her life is a testimony of God's goodness and the power of parents who refuse to lose hope.

Brittany was nonverbal until age six and had difficulty with social interaction and eye contact. She never learned to babble or crawl. Apraxia caused Brittany to struggle formulating the sounds of words and understanding verbal instructions. She was also unable to learn sign language due to her inability to plan and process motor tasks.

Cathy, her mother, shares, "When Brittany was hurt or felt ill, unlike most children, she refused hugs. I was the only person able to touch her physically without her experiencing a meltdown. She experienced many sensory issues. Brittany did not like loud music or music that would come out of a certain speaker in our house. She did not like balloons popping or fireworks. Brittany did not know how to tell us if she was sick. I am not sure if it was a language issue or if she did not understand what she was feeling. If she became overstimulated or had a sensory overload, Brittany's body would immediately tighten up."

At age three, Brittany was diagnosed on the autism spectrum with pervasive developmental disorder. Cathy was determined not to let a diagnosis limit Brittany. "I just expected her to do the same things as any other baby. It was just going to take her a little bit longer." Brittany received speech and language therapy with occupational therapy. She also participated in the program NACD to help her overcome apraxia which included vision therapy, sensory therapy, auditory processing programs, visual processing programs, and educational components. Brittany was in therapy six to seven hours a day.

Cathy decided to homeschool Brittany to help her learn social skills. As a young child, Brittany's only friend was her younger brother AJ, and they did everything together. When AJ's friends came over, she would interact with them, but only for a few minutes.

Cathy states, "Brittany played alongside AJ and his friends but never really interacted with them. She was in her own autistic land. Brittany was active in gymnastics and tae kwon do because AJ was in those sports, but she would isolate herself."

Until AJ played tennis. Suddenly a light came on for Brittany. Her mom says, "Tennis was a lifesaver—it helped her make friends and become a role model for other athletes."

When asked what life would be without tennis, Brittany quickly responds, "It would not be fun. I would not make new friends, and I would not compete. Tennis is my passion and helps me grow up to be a better person and athlete. I like to travel around the world playing tennis. I like the medals and trophies. I love everything about it."

Tennis became the gleam of dawn for Brittany and her parents. Of course there were regressions and struggles. Before a match, she needs help tying her shoes and putting her hair in a ponytail. But playing tennis caused a dramatic improvement in Brittany's gross and fine motor skills, visual perception, and processing skills which helped her to handle her emotions. Through tennis, Brittany is learning to adapt to situations she does not feel comfortable with and overcome life's obstacles. Brittany's greatest challenges to overcome are communication and change in routine—she still loves to escape into her room to stim during social gatherings.

Brittany brought home the gold in singles and doubles at the INAS World Tennis Championships and Special Olympics Florida State Championship in 2015. The next year, she competed in the Orlando United Double Tennis Open in a unified pair, which is two players where one has an intellectual disability and the other does not. Not only did she and her partner win gold, she was the only Special Olympics athlete invited to compete! At the 2018 Special Olympics USA Games, she won two gold medals. In March 2019, she won two silver medals at the Special Olympics World Games in Abu Dhabi.

Brittany is currently ranked first for female tennis players in the world for the Special Olympics and is a professional player. She has hit with legendary professional players like Andy Roddick and Bob Bryan, a winner of twenty-three Grand Slam titles. "It was so fun hitting with them at the Pro-Am tournament. Bob Bryan was so nice. We played doubles together. It was a great honor to play with him," Brittany shares.

Brittany travels around the world playing tennis. She has competed in seven countries: Greece, Australia, France, Dominican Republic, England, United Arab Emirates, and Ecuador. Australia is Brittany's favorite country. "I love the wildlife. Seeing kangaroos, wallabies, and adorable koalas. But most of all I love the tennis competition there."

The ability to laser focus on her single interest empowers Brittany to vigorously prepare for her matches. She does strength training three days a week and plays tennis five to six days a week for two to four hours. In her free time, Brittany volunteers at Dogs Unlimited and enjoys staying active in the pool and at the beaches in Orlando, Florida. She also loves spending time with her four dogs.

> "Every individual with autism is different and brings different talents and gifts to the world."

Cathy notes that following her child's passions and interests has led to new skills for Brittany, both physical and social. Cathy says, "I am still amazed at all the things Brittany has overcome. All young adults, with or without autism, deserve to be respected and embraced for themselves. They were created by God and are perfect exactly the way they are. Parents, let your child's light shine brightly so the world can see their talents and beautiful soul."

Brittany's goal is to keep improving her tennis skills and travel the world. Cathy shares, "We recently bought a café called Nature's Table to provide Brittany with steady employment. Brittany works the cash register and is learning to count money, talk to customers, and interact better with people."

Brittany encourages young adults with autism, "Believe in yourself and keep trying. I do not think any individual should be limited because of their disabilities. Autism is just a label and does not define a person. Every individual with autism is different and brings different talents and gifts to the world. I have overcome so much and continue to better myself each day on and off the court."

CLOSING THOUGHTS

During your family's journey with autism, there will be seasons of slow progress, and you'll feel discouraged. Remember to trust God, who brings on gradual growth. Everyone gets discouraged sometimes, but rather than adopting a spirit of complaint, make a conscious effort to praise God in the midst of therapies and your tedious schedule. You'll find it makes a difference in both your and your child's attitudes.

Don't allow autism to drain your energy. Relax, stay calm, and enjoy the first gleam of dawn because it points to great things to come.

PRAYER AND MEDITATION

Prayer

As the first gleam of dawn welcomes a fresh day with new opportunities, so, Father, shine your light on my path—let me see the spark in my child's interests which leads to progress in speech and social interaction. When days are difficult, remind me of the progress we've made in the past. And help me, Lord, to pay close attention to my child's progress so that I recognize even the smallest of achievements. Nehemiah 8:10 calls for us to not be sad, but to remember that "the joy of the LORD is your strength." Thank you for your joy and your strength. Amen.

Meditation

May the God of hope fill you with all joy and peace as you trust in him, so that you may overflow with hope by the power of the Holy Spirit. (Romans 15:13)

Do not grieve, for the joy of the LORD is your strength. (Nehemiah 8:10)

Chapter 15

Empowerment for Parenting Endurance

By perseverance, the snail reached the ark.
—CHARLES SPURGEON

*You need to persevere so that when you have done the will of
God, you will receive what he has promised. For, "In just a little
while, he who is coming will come and will not delay."*
—HEBREWS 10:36–37

RAISING CHILDREN CAN easily drain all your power and motivation, especially raising a child with autism or other disabilities. When my daughter, Makayla, has the flu and continually cries, "I want my mommy," I feel exhausted and want my mommy too.

If we're continually hit with life's difficulties, it's a struggle to love others and maintain patience. Ultimately we experience frustration, lose our joy, and dread life. Jesus fully recognized this downward spiral when he said, "The love of most will grow cold" (Matthew 24:12). But he also said, "Stand firm, and you will win life" (Luke 21:19). He's given us the way to go from cold frustration to joy and life. Standing firm is a conscious choice on our part, and in order to stand firm, we must find balance. Did you know that Jesus instilled some balance in his life? In Mark 4:35–40, we see how Jesus took time to rest. He showed up when a crisis was at hand, but prior to that, he was sleeping, because he was human and had the same need for rest that we do. All four gospels—Matthew, Mark, Luke, and John—give multiple accounts of Jesus seeking solitude and prayer time with the Father. Yes, Jesus had a hugely important job to do, and yet he took time to care for his mental, emotional, spiritual, and physical health. We need to follow his example and make time to take care of our mental, emotional, spiritual, and physical health too.

While self-care can look different for each person, here are a few suggestions that may work to help you find the balance to stand firm.

1. Find and do things you enjoy.

You can bring your child with you to do things you enjoy. This will expose them to new smells and activities, and you might find that your child actually enjoys them too. Of course, be prepared for them not to enjoy them as much as you do. As a family we find it relaxing to go to the swimming pool in the summer and to walk the indoor mall in the winter.

During fun downtime, you can visit new places. I love to google cool places in Michigan and visit them. One of my favorite places to travel nearby is Frankenmuth, a German town that is famous for its Christmas store. Fun mini trips do not have to be expensive. You can visit many local nature parks for free and many cities have free fun events. One city near our home has a free outdoor movie night in the summer. This relaxing time can help us collect our thoughts and regain strength.

2. Make downtime to release stress.

Build in time to breathe and listen to birds. Take a short walk outside, talk to a friend on the phone, prepare a meal to celebrate life. For downtime, my mom would go on nature walks in the woods. Once a year, she would attend a women's retreat with friends from church. For downtime I like to go for a short three-mile run or watch a documentary film. There are documentaries on almost every subject imaginable, and you might learn about a topic or issue that inspires you.

Find a quiet place to let your mind reflect on life. When we're deep in work routines, it can be hard to tear ourselves away from immediate tasks. By removing ourselves from these day-to-day stressors, we can daydream and enjoy the moment.

> ## Remember to take self-care turns with your spouse or other caregivers to give each other a break.

When I am stressed from working long hours at the hospital, I treat myself to a good meal. A new seafood entrée hits the spot or dinner at a nice Italian restaurant. Also remember to take self-care turns with your spouse or other caregivers to give each other a break. Every human needs downtime; it's necessary to keep our strength and maintain balance . . . and our sanity.

3. Take advantage of programs at local organizations.

Structured organizations can provide temporary relief and enable you to take a much-needed break from the demands of caregiving. Find a local church that provides respite care or an autism organization that offers parents a night out. For example, a church near our home has a Christmas party for special needs families. This event helps families to connect with other special needs families and enjoy the holiday season. Or consider how a church special needs program can help you connect with volunteers who can provide relief time for your dentist or doctor appointments.

Autism Support and Resource Center in Genesee County, Michigan, has Power Camp. This is a five-day day camp for individuals with autism, and the staff is professionally trained. You can drop off your camper and know that she will be safe and have a fun day.

When is the last time you and your spouse went on a date? Just the two of you? I can't stress enough the importance of scheduling regular date nights with your spouse. If family isn't an option to care for your child, find a sitter who understands your child and can develop a relationship with him or her. Local college students studying ABA therapy are a great place to look. Contact local colleges and inquire about hiring students with an educational background in autism. It will give you peace of mind to go do something for yourself or with your spouse, knowing that your child is secure and safe. Rest and refreshment will empower you to care for your family.

Steve and Anne Aurand, the parents of Walker, a young adult with Asperger's, discovered joy and self-care through hockey. Through hockey and his parent's love, Walker Aurand's life became a testimony of transforming adversity into opportunity. Walker's love for the game caused him to refuse to let autism hold him back from accomplishing his dream of playing Division I college hockey.

Walker Aurand: The First ACHA Division I Hockey Player with Autism

Steve and Anne Aurand, to relax and enjoy self-care time, took their sons regularly to the ice rink.[1] Years later, hockey and ice skating were instrumental for their son with Asperger's to learn social skills and achieve college success.

Basic skills like tying shoes, writing, and interacting with friends were extremely difficult for Walker Aurand. But on the ice, Walker was a natural and began skating at only two years old. When his dad, Steve, took him to the rink at Davenport University in Grand Rapids, Michigan, for open skate, he was astonished to see his two-year-old son skating without any training. Walker shares, "When my parents took hold of my hand on the ice, after five minutes I let go, looked back at them, and said, 'I'm good. I can do this by myself.' Whenever I step on the ice, I feel clarity. My worries and insecurities disappear."

Walker's parents first realized something was unique about their son when he was three months old. While he was lying on the living room floor, his dad leaned over him and said, "Hi, buddy," and Walker clearly responded, "Hi."

Walker's parents were astonished. Anne recalls, "I didn't know whether to be happy or go, 'Oh my gosh, who does that?'"

There were other surprises while raising Walker. Anne and Steve noticed the sound of the microwave door opening or Velcro ripping caused their son to have meltdowns. He also struggled to go to sleep or eat. Issues with changes in routine and transitions, weak fine motor skills, and sensory issues caused Walker to be diagnosed with autism at the age of three.

Walker shares his experience with autism. "I was unable to hold a pencil the right way as a child—it was difficult to read words all the way through and read quickly. Learning to tie my shoes was a pain. Change in routines would almost always make me feel thrown off. I had difficultly picking up on sarcasm and social cues."

As a child, Walker received speech, vision, and occupational therapy. At the age of eight, his parents told him he had autism. They discovered ways to help him stay calm. When he felt overwhelmed physically, they would use a cleaning brush to gently brush his arms and legs, or swing him in a blanket to bring relief. Certain smells, like cinnamon, enabled Walker's brain to feel more organized.

"I'm lucky to have a mother who is a speech pathologist and worked with kids like me—this really helped me overcome some of the challenges. My parents made many sacrifices. I can't begin to say how much they have done. They've given me everything. My dad was my coach, and he took me to my games early in the morning. My mom always was patient with me in my schoolwork and helped me learn to understand the social environment around me. I'm so lucky to have the parents I have— they always wanted the best for me. I wouldn't be the person I am today without their love and support."

Walker loved playing sports with his younger brother, Brendan, and his parents encouraged him to play hockey. "My parents noticed when I was little, I was happy on the ice. I had good hand-eye coordination, and I can skate well. I like hockey because it is a sport that brings people together. It also highlights my capabilities and athletic talent. Hockey gives me a rush of adrenaline and a chance to be on a winning team."

Walker describes hockey as therapeutic and freeing to both mind and body. "When you're on the ice, you almost feel like you can fly."

One of the challenges he had to overcome was sarcasm in the locker room. "I learned to adapt to the locker room environment. My brother Brendan played high school hockey with me and helped me figure out sarcasm and when I was being teased. I'm very confident in myself. I believe a lot of it has to do with all the hardships I've had to overcome. I wouldn't trade those hardships because they've helped me become who I am."

Steve talked a bit about Walker's competitive nature, which has been with him since he was young. During his first year playing, whenever his team lost, Walker would have a meltdown. He would get so upset, in fact, that he couldn't gain control of himself to finish the game.

A few games, Steve had to carry his son out by his jersey, kicking and screaming, arms flailing through the air with him shouting, "No, I want to win! No, you can't take me off the ice!"

"Yes we can, son," Steve would calmly respond.

"I have autism, but autism doesn't have me."

Anne and Steve used hockey as a therapy to teach Walker to spell. They would take unbreakable plates and write a letter on each one. Then they would hang the letter plates from the net, spelling out a word. He would shoot at each letter as they rehearsed the letters and the word they spelled. C-A-T, cat. P-A-N, pan. While this might not work for every child, it helped Walker. Anne shares, "He eventually learned to read through some of that and sound things out, and it became his sensory therapy with the crashing and burning on the ice. It was kind of a multipurpose thing, and, you know, the bottom line is he really, really loved it."[2]

By the end of the second grade, Walker was a good speller and had received hundreds of hours of therapies, which was very time-consuming for his family. Playing hockey empowered Walker to learn social skills and gain self-confidence. "The number of friends I've made over my life is something that I'll never forget. Some of my best friends now are people from hockey that I've met growing up. I'll cherish those friendships forever, and I'll never forget how much my friends and family mean to me. I think hockey has taught me how to react to different situations and to become stronger in difficult times through my friendships."

During Walker's senior year of high school, his English teacher assigned a paper that asked students to share one way they could change the world. He decided to finally let his peers know about his autism. In Walker's essay, he shares, "I have autism, but autism doesn't have me."

A family friend, who is an artist, asked Walker if she could paint his portrait and include a quote from his essay to exhibit at ArtPrize in Grand Rapids, Michigan. The international art competition attracts nearly half a million attendees every year. After a week of contemplating, Walker agreed to reveal his autism to the world.

The day of the exhibition, Walker returned from school "freaked out." He told his mom, "All these kids saw my painting at ArtPrize. My phone is blowing up. I bet I have 150 texts: 'Is that you, Walker?' 'Is that you, Walker?' Mom, I didn't know I had friends." She asked how he felt about it. "I've decided it's okay," Walker replied.

After high school, Walker played a season of hockey for Dells Ducks of the Minnesota Junior Hockey League. He packed his belongings and moved six hours away to Dells, Wisconsin, to play hockey for the next eight months with people he had never met.

Walker shares his experience of being away from home and living with a billet family—a family who invites junior players into their homes to be a part of their family during the hockey season. "I was fortunate to be able to play and live with one of my best friends from high school which made the transition to Dells easier for both of us. Before I left, my parents talked to my coach and billet family to let them know that I had autism and explain what it was. I never expected any special treatment because of my autism, but we felt it was important for them both to know this about me."

Walker noted that his parents helped him get ready for the summer by teaching him the skills of self-advocating and setting up his own routine. Being on the spectrum, Walker finds routine extremely important. They taught him all of the skills necessary to manage his own daily needs.

"While I enjoyed my time with the Ducks, a part of me really missed home and seeing all my friends. It was nice not having to worry about school during the week, but when I would see someone I knew from back home really enjoying their college experience, a part of me felt like I was missing out on something.

"After playing a year of junior hockey in Wisconsin for the Dells Ducks, I made the decision to go to Davenport because I wanted my parents to be able to see me play, and I wanted to be closer to home. My connection with the coaching staff and memories of the team as a child made DU an easy pick. It's kind of come full circle. My dad was the goalie coach for the Davenport University program when it first began, so I knew the program well."

Walker Aurand wears the #55 jersey and is one of the top defensemen on Davenport University's ACHA Division I Hockey Team. Walker has taken his adversities with autism and turned them into an advantage. "I am obsessive and as a result, I have a good work ethic and tend to be a perfectionist. I like to keep improving and that makes me work extremely hard to correct my mistakes and just keep on getting better at this sport."

Walker is now pursuing a degree in marketing and desires a career in sports media as a blogger or analyst. He also would love to coach hockey. "My more immediate goal is to win Davenport a national championship," Walker exclaims.

Entering his senior year, Walker reflects on his journey. "College has given me the opportunity to grow through different experiences and figure out who I am. My hockey teammates are very accepting and have been there for me. I am truly blessed with these teammates. They make me a better player. They are the reason I am excited to come to the rink every day."

As an autism advocate, Walker states, "I'm someone who young kids with similar disabilities can look up to and that means more to me than any award or win. Hockey has given me a platform to be an advocate for people with disabilities and it's helped me to try to improve the lives of those around me. I am grateful for that."

Walker encourages young adults with autism: "Never be afraid of change or new things and don't be afraid to fail because failure is a part of life. Life's not easy, but if we try hard enough, we can turn adversity to our advantage. Above all else, have conviction in who you are, find what you are passionate about, and go for it."

Because Steve and Anne took the time to practice self-care, and their children enjoyed the same activity, Walker's gift for and love of hockey was discovered. And Steve and Anne got to relax and refresh a bit.

CLOSING THOUGHTS

Maybe you need to take a break and enjoy some downtime. Go for a walk, prepare a good meal, or listen to peaceful music. Relax; life is short. Self-care—giving focused attention to mental, emotional, spiritual, and physical health—will help you to stand firm in times of adversity and help you to enjoy life again.

PRAYER AND MEDITATION

Prayer

Lord, I go through times of focusing so intently on my child that I forget to stop and refresh myself. Please help me to be mindful of taking breaks and finding ways to relax. Help me to slow down and enjoy the moment. Please provide resources for respite so I can relax and rejuvenate. Focus my mind on your peace and love. Grant me rest when I am weary. Amen.

Meditation

> I am convinced that neither death nor life, neither angels nor demons, neither the present nor the future, nor any powers, neither height nor depth, nor anything else in all creation, will be able to separate us from the love of God that is in Christ Jesus our Lord. (Romans 8:38–39)

> Then, because so many people were coming and going that they did not even have a chance to eat, he said to them, "Come with me by yourselves to a quiet place and get some rest." (Mark 6:31)

P A R T   4

Resting in God

Chapter 16

Soaring as Eagles

As a child who was severely bullied, I felt like a turkey on
Thanksgiving: fearful of the massacre to come. However, with
God's grace and power, I have learned to soar like an eagle.

—Ron Sandison

He gives strength to the weary and increases the power of the
weak. Even youths grow tired and weary, and young men
stumble and fall; but those who hope in the Lord will renew
their strength. They will soar on wings like eagles; they will run
and not grow weary, they will walk and not be faint.

—Isaiah 40:29–31

There is no doubt that parenting a child with autism requires God's wisdom and strength. But you don't have to do it alone. As God proclaimed to Moses in Exodus 19:4, "You yourselves have seen what I did to Egypt, and how I carried you on eagles' wings and brought you to myself." While you likely aren't in literal slavery or wandering in a desert like the Israelites, you might feel similarly to them—trapped and desperate. God promises he will carry us on eagles' wings and bring us to himself. But what does that mean for us?

The Bible often uses the image of the eagle to symbolize the strength, grace, and provision God gives his people. Just like God delivered miracles and provisions for the Israelites, and Moses got to know the heart of God and his passions, God promises to provide for and draw near to you too. It may not look the way you hope it will, but he "is able to do immeasurably more than all we ask or imagine" (Ephesians 3:20).

God Is Always Present and Knows What You Need

My daughter, Makayla, loves to play hide-and-seek. Her favorite hiding spot is under the covers in our bed with her stuffed animals. She is easy to find because you can hear her joyfully laughing as you enter the room. I play along, hiding in the closet, and Makayla always calls out, "I know you're here."

As parents of children on the spectrum, we know that it sometimes feels like God is hiding from us, not as part of a game but out of neglect or inability to do what we feel we need to have done. But really, life is much more like my fun hide-and-seek game with Makayla than we may realize. Psalm 91:4 shares that God "will cover you with his feathers, and under his wings you will find refuge; his faithfulness will be your shield and rampart." God is always present and always knows where we are and what we need.

But knowing these facts doesn't always feel helpful in the middle of a crisis. So what's an overwhelmed parent to do?

1. Give your worries to Jesus.

In the Bible in the book of Luke, Martha also experienced life's overload moments and complained about it to Jesus:

> As Jesus and his disciples were on their way, he came to a village where a woman named Martha opened her home to him. She had a sister called Mary, who sat at the Lord's feet listening to what he said. But Martha was distracted by all the preparations that had to be made. She came to him and asked, "Lord, don't

you care that my sister has left me to do the work by myself? Tell her to help me!"

"Martha, Martha," the Lord answered, "you are worried and upset about many things, but few things are needed—or indeed only one. Mary has chosen what is better, and it will not be taken away from her." (10:38–42)

When Martha was overwhelmed, she went to Jesus. That is always the first step. When God's presence seems absent, we need to step away from our busywork and the noise around us and pray for God to reveal himself.

2. Trust God to provide for your needs.

Jesus promises to provide for our needs and, in turn, we're not to worry.

Therefore I tell you, do not worry about your life, what you will eat or drink; or about your body, what you will wear. Is not life more than food, and the body more than clothes? Look at the birds of the air; they do not sow or reap or store away in barns, and yet your heavenly Father feeds them. Are you not much more valuable than they? . . .

But seek first his kingdom and his righteousness, and all these things will be given to you as well. Therefore do not worry about tomorrow, for tomorrow will worry about itself. Each day has enough trouble of its own. (Matthew 6:25–26, 33–34)

The greatest lesson my parents taught me is to trust God and place my worries in the hands of Jesus. My first semester of seminary, I felt overwhelmed taking a full course load and biblical Greek. I called my dad and said, "Please pray for me. I am terrified that I won't be able to pass all my classes and comprehend Greek."

My dad replied, "Did God call you to get your Master of Divinity?"

"Yes."

"Don't worry. Place your classes in Jesus's hands. Where God guides, he will provide."

I soon discovered autism was the perfect gift for learning Greek. Unlike other languages, Greek is taught visually instead of phonetically. Because I am a visual learner, I was able to master biblical Greek and translate two-thirds of the New Testament without trouble.

3. Accept Jesus's invitation to rest.

If we look back at the passage in Luke where Martha complains to Jesus, we might expect Jesus to give Martha a time-out for whining. But he doesn't. Jesus responds with compassion. In following Jesus, we need to be careful we don't keep ourselves so busy working for the Lord that there's no time to simply be with the Lord.

> If you're feeling overwhelmed,
> talk to God about it.

Jesus notes that Martha feels frantic and worried, and then he invites her to rest.

If you're feeling overwhelmed, talk to God about it, do what you can to step back, and spend some time seeing what God is doing around you. Try to find some balance.

4. Make time to enjoy your family.

Having a child with autism doesn't make it easy to rest. One of the best things you can do is to find ways to have fun with your family. This releases you from the isolation autism can bring and helps your child develop new skills and friendships.

My parents made sure my brothers and I were involved in many activities including Cub Scouts, YMCA, karate, and church youth groups. These programs provided bonding time with our family, positive role models, a sense of independence, and lifelong friendships, as well as persistence and tenacity.

Julie Hornok shares her insight on helping children discover new activities:

When Lizzie was younger, she had a really hard time doing anything that wasn't in her routine. We found that making a detailed social story with real pictures helped prepare her and even allowed her to look forward to new activities. I would go before each new activity and take pictures and map out exactly what her time would be like to decrease any anxiety the new activity would cause. The more she tried new things, the easier it was. I was able to do less and less detailed social stories as time went on, and now we don't need to use them at all. Consistency and slowly pulling back on the support as your child is more and more capable is key.[1]

My favorite childhood memories are family events. I still remember going to the zoo with my mom and my brother Chuckie, watching prairie dogs eat dandelions while the tigers slept. I learned to socialize by enjoying fun activities and asking questions. And my parents were able to relax just a bit.

5. Discover God's hidden provision in the wilderness.

In the seasons of life when we feel discouraged and spiritually dry, God provides us with grace and strength to grow spiritually. I refer to these seasons as "the wilderness" because we feel barren and lost, but rest assured that God is renewing our strength. Psalm 103:5 says that the Lord "satisfies your desires with good things so that your youth is renewed like the eagle's."

> When we feel abandoned in the wilderness, we must remember that God is with us, sending his provision.

Let's consider the Old Testament prophet Elijah. Even Elijah experienced seasons in the wilderness, requiring him to trust God and overcome his fears. Elijah pronounced three years of famine in Canaan due to King Ahab and his wife Jezebel's disobedience to God. The king and queen did not like this news and wanted to kill Elijah, so God told him to escape to the desert. The Lord instructed him to go down to Kerith Ravine and drink from the brook. He was told the ravens would feed him (1 Kings 17:4), and he remained there until the brook dried up from the drought. Let's be clear. Elijah was in a desert with no food or water, and the king and queen were trying to kill him. He's in as dark a place as a human can be. And God sends ravens.

If you've ever seen an eagle in the wild, you realize just how majestic these animals truly are. Ravens, on the other hand, are common and, frankly, pretty unimpressive scavengers. Ironically, the raven is the very bird God chooses to feed bread and meat to Elijah (see 1 Kings 17). Three valuable lessons can be learned by God's choice of bird.

1. *God can bless us in any circumstance.* God can use anything, even the most common and unimpressive, to feed and bless us. He is not limited by our circumstances or environment. In the desert, Isaac was able to reap a hundred times as much as his usual crop because the Lord had blessed him (Genesis 26:12).
2. *God provides in our wilderness.* Even though it doesn't feel like it, we are blessed in the wilderness seasons when God is our only source of provision. If this common and unimpressive bird fed Elijah, how much more should Elijah, a prophet of God himself, have fed and cared for the people of Israel, winning them over to follow God? As for Elijah, wilderness seasons allow us to reflect and learn compassion from God's divine wisdom.
3. *God offers growth in the wilderness.* The wilderness seasons refine us to be a blessing to other families who have children with autism. After Elijah's desert experience, he traveled to Zarephath where he spent three years in refinement learning mercy and compassion. He then returned to Israel to confront evil and win the Israelites back to God. God's refining teaches us to cease relying on our natural strength and instead rely on his grace.

During the Great Recession of 2005, I went through a wilderness season of underemployment and unemployment. When I experienced financial hardship, I learned to pray and trust God for my provision. God was refining my heart to have compassion for individuals with autism who also struggle with employment. In 2016, I founded Spectrum Inclusion, which empowers young adults with disabilities to gain independence and employment. The founding of this organization has given me empathy for those struggling with employment and a desire to see them succeed.

When we feel abandoned in the wilderness, we must remember that God is with us, sending his provision. Even people of great faith and good deeds experience doubt and paralyzing fear, often in the midst of loneliness, dejection, and silence. The Bible teaches that Elijah was a human, just like us (James 5:17). It's reassuring to know we're in good company.

Erik N. Weber, an attorney with autism, is a perfect illustration about discovering the power to soar as an eagle by Christ's power and grace. He shares, "Knowing God has a plan for our lives gives us hope that no challenge is too great." Erik's incredible story has been featured on NBC 7 San Diego.

Erik Weber: Reaching New Heights

Erik Weber's development appeared typical until he reached two and a half years old; after experiencing a high fever, he began to regress rapidly.[2] At that time Erik's mother, Sandy, noticed he ceased to respond to her voice and failed to maintain proper eye contact. Afraid she was losing her son, Sandy had Erik tested. Neurological specialists diagnosed her beautiful, brown-eyed, three-year-old son as autistic with mental retardation. When Erik was five, doctors warned his parents his autism was so severe, he would likely not progress past the cognitive level of an eighteen-month-old child. It was recommended that he be institutionalized.

Sandy was determined to empower her son to overcome his disabilities, so she went to the one person she knew could help. Erik states, "My mom prayed continually for God's guidance for my life. A teaching method she implemented was videotaping my behavior and playing it back to me because I was a visual learner. She also used Picture Exchange Communication System Cards. I would hand my mom the card for the things I wanted."

Erik's special interests as a child were Thomas the Train and NASCAR, and his mom used these interests to help him in his language development and social skills.

Like Martha, Sandy went to God and complained about the situation, and then Sandy sought help. She encourages parents who have a child with special needs to "grieve the loss of the perfect child so that you can embrace the child that you have and maximize whatever his or her potential will be."

Erik began to speak at age seven and had dysgraphia—extreme difficulty with handwriting. He also had tactile sensory issues, hating to be touched. When he received a shot at the doctor's office, Erik would scream before the needle even pricked his skin.

Sandy encouraged Erik's faith in Christ, and as a young child, he gave his heart to Jesus. Erik recalls one defining moment in his faith: "As a young child, my mom would play the song *All We Like Sheep*, and I would sing along, praising Jesus for his goodness."

One area that God gave Sandy a hidden provision was the daughter of Erik's preschool teacher. Erik shares, "Mom believed the daughter of my preschool teacher was the only person who would be able to help me start to talk, since she was able to involve me in activities I wouldn't have been able to do otherwise." Because of their friendship, Sandy decided to keep Erik in preschool for a few extra years.

Sandy's prayers were answered. The young girl encouraged Erik to express himself with language, helping to free him from his isolated world. From third grade through high school, Erik attended a private school designed to help children with disabilities achieve independence and success. By seventh grade, Erik was so advanced in his academics that he skipped eighth grade and was able to graduate from high school a year early, in 2006. As for this close friend, she graduated from college with a degree in occupational therapy so she can help children with special needs. The two still share a close bond.

While Erik was attending grade school, his father passed away. Soon after, his mother encouraged him to compete in the Special Olympics, because she wanted her son to have positive role models and develop self-esteem. Special Olympics helped Erik to soar to new heights. Erik shares,

"I have won 139 Special Olympics medals, including 117 gold medals. I hope to become a Special Olympics track-and-field coach. I love to run because I feel the wind against my face, my anxiety is reduced, and most importantly, it reminds me of being a kid riding on the back of my father's motorcycle."

Special Olympics provided an environment for Erik to develop friendships, confidence, and both physical and mental endurance. Years later, these qualities were instrumental in helping him pass the California bar exam.

Erik mentors middle school students with attention deficit hyperactivity disorder and autism who are training to run in the Special Olympics. "My drive is to help others with 'diffabilities' to be champions," Erik explains.

Erik was able to develop social skills with his savant ability to memorize and quote famous comedians, even perfectly mimicking their voices and mannerisms. Some of Erik's favorites include Kevin Hart, Will Ferrell, Robin Williams, and Steve Harvey. Erik shares, "While in college, for an icebreaker when meeting girls, I'd ask, 'Who's your favorite comedian?' After the girl replied, I would proceed to impersonate her favorite comedian. If I was lucky, I would get a kiss on the cheek for my performance."

In 2009, Erik earned a bachelor's degree in International Development Studies with a 3.9 GPA from Point Loma Nazarene University. Next, he earned a master's degree in Public Administration from San Diego State University with a 3.7 GPA.

When NBC San Diego interviewed Erik about being accepted to law school, he responded, "People call me the trailblazer, the icon, but I'm an ordinary person doing extraordinary things." In May 2015, he became the first Cal Western School of Law student with autism to pass the California bar exam, passing it on his first try.

Erik jokes, "The doctors told my parents to put me in an institution and that turned out to be law school. Autism has helped me as an attorney to be honest, do the right thing, and put my clients first."

Erik declares, "God is using me as an example of what people with special needs can do. I hope to practice special education law full-time so

I can help others like me to find their voice and pursue their potential." As Jeremiah 22:16 says, "'He defended the cause of the poor and needy, and so all went well. Is that not what it means to know me?' declares the LORD."

Erik spent much of 2020 training for the 2020 Big Sur International Marathon and running 6.5 miles a day, while practicing special education law, as God opened doors for him as a lawyer.

CLOSING THOUGHTS

Job 39:27 says, "Does the eagle soar at your command and build its nest on high?" No, we're not in control of the universe. God empowers us by his fuel of grace and love to soar like eagles and build godly families. Our response is to bring our worries to Jesus and allow him to reveal his hidden provisions. Psalm 63:7–8 says, "Because You have been my help, therefore in the shadow of Your wings I will rejoice. My soul follows close behind You; Your right hand upholds me" (NKJV).

PRAYER AND MEDITATION

Prayer

God, by your grace and love, empower me to soar like the eagle. Give me patience and faith to love and care for my family. Open my eyes to see your gracious provision during the wilderness seasons when I feel alone and afraid. Cover and protect me in the shadow of your wing and empower me to be a blessing. Amen.

Meditation

And I will give you treasures hidden in the darkness—secret riches. I will do this so you may know that I am the LORD, the God of Israel, the one who calls you by name. (Isaiah 45:3 NLT)

Jesus often withdrew to lonely places and prayed. (Luke 5:16)

Chapter 17

God's Got This

The Christian . . . trusts [God] where he cannot trace him,
looks up to him in the darkest hour, and believes that all is well.

—CHARLES SPURGEON

And we know that in all things God works for the good
of those who love him, who have been called
according to his purpose.

—ROMANS 8:28

YOU'VE LIKELY HEARD some version of this old story over the years.

A man walks into a bar and says to the bartender, "Do you want to see something amazing?"

"Yes," the bartender replies.

The man crosses to a piano, sets a frog on the keyboard, and the frog begins to jam.

"Wow!" the bartender exclaims.

"Do you want to see something even more spectacular?"

"Of course!"

The man places a white mouse next to the frog, and the mouse sings and dances while the frog plays the piano. A crowd gathers around the man and his amphibian-rodent band.

"I'll give you a hundred dollars for that singing mouse," someone in the crowd shouts.

"Sure," says the man.

The man relinquishes the white mouse, accepts the hundred dollar bill, and as he turns to leave, the bartender just shakes his head. "You're a fool. You could've made millions with the frog and mouse act in Hollywood."

The man winks and says, "I forgot to tell the buyer one important detail. The frog is a ventriloquist."

Throughout my journey, I have often felt much like the white mouse; I am not worth much alone and have little control of where I go. My success has been dependent on God's strength and grace. He is, in a sense, my ventriloquist. I suspect that's true of most people, but from my view on the spectrum, that truth is even stronger.

God Moments

My friend Karla Barnett, who is the founder of Dynamic Kids and has a son with autism, gave me a plastic wristband with the words "God's Got This." I love this declaration of faith. God *is* in control, and he will give us wisdom and guidance in raising our children. He will also send people along our path to bless us and our families.

The keys to my success all have one thing in common: God moments, or as the bracelet states, "God's Got This." Even the secular community acknowledges the concept of "God moments," only they refer to them as luck or karma: preparation meeting opportunity. God moments consist of seemingly random events and painful life experiences masterfully woven together by God to create a beautiful work of art—that's my life and it's your life. We were "created in Christ Jesus to do good works, which God prepared in advance for us to do" (Ephesians 2:10).

Steve Jobs, the founder of Apple, described God moments from a secular perspective when he said, "You can't connect the dots looking forward; you can only connect them looking backward. So you have to trust that the dots will somehow connect in your future. You have to trust in something—your gut, destiny, life, karma, whatever."[1]

Philip Yancey, from a Christian perspective, asks, "What is faith, after all, but believing in advance what will only make sense in reverse?"[2]

Scratch board art is an excellent metaphor for God's ability to work in our children's lives and transform our darkness and pain for his glory. Oral Roberts University has a campus student fun day. During their event, they have a professional artist create scratch board art. This art is created by spraying five layers of different paint colors onto a board, topped by a coating of black, and then carving out of the darkness. The result is a masterful panoply painting.

When I attended this event, the artist made me a scratch board art plaque of a futuristic city with bluish green waterfalls and a red moon. In redemption, like the scratch board art, Christ cuts through our layers of failures, sins, and pains—the blackness—and transforms them for his glory—the beautiful hidden colors showing through. In your dark hours—trying to choose the right therapies to help your child or feeling overwhelmed about your child's future—God is creating light out of the darkness.

God continues to create beauty out of darkness.

In *The Message* paraphrase of the Bible, Genesis 1:1–2 describes God's power to transform darkness into light: "First this: God created the Heavens and Earth—all you see, all you don't see. Earth was a soup of nothingness, a bottomless emptiness, an inky blackness. God's Spirit brooded like a bird above the watery abyss."[3] And from that darkness God created not only brilliant light but all the beauty contained in our world. And he didn't stop at creation. To this day God continues to create beauty out of darkness.

Pastor Jason Hague describes the brokenness and beauty in our world: "Our world, then, will never be one-dimensional. Here, victory and defeat comingle. Here, weddings and funerals occur under the same roof. The world is full of both beauty and brokenness, of question marks and exclamation points, of smooth roads and potholes. Tension and mystery are sewn into the tapestry of creation, and they will last to the end of the age."[4]

God's Guidance and Wisdom

I owe much of my success to my mom. But she would say God used her to create God moments for me. As a child, I was unable to learn phonetically and had dyslexia, writing my name and other words backward. Following the teaching in James 1:5 to pray for wisdom, my mom prayed, "Holy Spirit, guide me and give me wisdom in teaching my son to read, write, and comprehend information."

The Holy Spirit spoke to my mom's heart and said, "Ron's love for animals and art can unlock his ability to learn how to read and write and develop social skills." It was a God moment that opened up an enormous avenue for my mom to teach me. When I was five years old, I dictated short fictional animal stories to my mom; she would write the stories in spiral notebooks and then have me rewrite the stories. Within two years of learning visually, the dyslexia was gone.

She taught me social skills using Chatter the Squirrel's letters. Chatter was an imaginary talking squirrel my mom invented to teach me. Each week, I received a handwritten letter in the mail from Chatter the Squirrel, teaching me new social skills such as active listening, good eye-contact, and tips on developing friendships.

Here's an example of a letter from Chatter, written back in 1982 (I still have them all):

> Dear Ronnie,
>   This is my new friend, Scamper. She came and stayed with me just recently. She is also friends with Bushy Tail. What I like about her is her peacefulness. She is a great <u>listener</u>. She carefully listens to all my chatter. She loves Jesus and shares with other squirrels in need. She has a shine in her eyes and loves to smile. I love my friend Scamper.
>
> Your friend, Chatter

Notice in my mom's letter from Chatter the Squirrel, the word *listener* is underlined. She underlined it for emphasis, because those of us on the spectrum tend to have difficulty listening to others. Dr. O. Ivar Lovaas, a pioneer in ABA therapy, said, "If they can't learn the way we teach, we teach the way they learn."[5] And it was my mom's prayer that opened a way for God to reveal an insight for my good.

Because my mom found ways for me to learn, I was able to attend middle school and high school with minimum accommodations. My parents paid for me to be tutored all throughout those years. These tutors were able to connect with me on a personal level and provided rewards for hard work, creating a desire to learn. Tutoring in math, reading, and English prepared me for the rigorous academics of college. The English tutoring was instrumental in giving me the ability to write and publish my first book, *A Parent's Guide to Autism*.

But it isn't just schooling where people on the spectrum struggle. Autism causes the executive functioning of my brain to have great difficulty with making important decisions; it took me two years to decide to purchase my 2005 Saturn Ion after my Geo Prizm died at 250,000 miles.

With my neurological wiring, choosing the right college or university felt impossible. It took a God moment; I was reading a random book and the author mentioned that her daughter attended Oral Roberts University. The Holy Spirit spoke to my heart and said, "Ron, I have called you to go to ORU." I was scared to death to travel 950 miles away from home to go to college in Tulsa, Oklahoma. My dad helped make the transition smoother by traveling with me to ORU during their college weekend to meet the students and faculty.

My freshman year of college, I first attended Michigan Christian College (now Rochester University) on an athletic scholarship for track and cross-country. When I graduated high school, my GPA was only a 2.5, but by attending Michigan Christian College, I was able to get my GPA up to a 3.9 and receive an academic scholarship to ORU. God connected the dots of athletics with academics. And by going away to college, I gained independence from my mom and dad.

Following God's Call

Today I am a husband, father, and a successful speaker and author. But you wouldn't know that from where I started.

Life certainly didn't make sense for me for a long while, just as it may not make sense for you and your child right now. But God has all of eternity to display his faithfulness. Lamentations 3:22–23 says, "Because of the LORD's great love we are not consumed, for his compassions never fail. They are new every morning; great is your faithfulness."

My employment history can best be described by a T-shirt I own. The shirt has a cartoon toothbrush with eyes saying, "I hate my job," to a roll of toilet paper, who replies, "Oh, please."

In 2005, I found myself unemployed and unable to find stable employment for three years. I was previously employed full-time at a large church in one town and part-time as a youth pastor at a church in another town. Due to the downfall in Michigan's economy and recession, I was let go from both churches—in the same week, no less!

For the next three years, I experienced unsteady employment, working four months at a skateboard shop for $5.25 an hour, five months at a moving company, and the remainder of the time as a youth specialist with at-risk youth. I felt confused and hurt. I began questioning, "Where are you, God? What have I done to find myself in this dark predicament?"

Even in the midst of refining, God still faithfully opened doors for me to minister and speak his Word. I found inspiration in Romans 8:28, "And we know that in all things God works for the good of those who love him, who have been called according to his purpose." My God moments journal entry for April 13, 2006, states: "Work on your people skills and pray for God to develop people skills in you." I also listed in my journal seven methods to improve my people skills.

1. Seek first to understand, then to be understood.
2. No monotone—Ron, you sound like a robot.
3. Timing of words. Proverb 15:23, "A person finds joy in giving an apt reply—and how good is a timely word!"
4. Have eye contact when talking to people.

5. Pronounce "Th" and "L" words by using the proper tongue movements.

6. Pray and seek the Lord.

7. Develop a strategy for people skills by imitating friends who have those skills.

During this trial, God was preparing me to be the Ron you see today. King Solomon said, "Remove the impurities from silver, and the sterling will be ready for the silversmith" (Proverbs 25:4 NLT). I was nearing the completion of my three years of darkness, though I didn't know it at the time. After a church service one Sunday, a congregant gave me a piece of paper with a handwritten message and told me that he believed the message was for me. The note stated, "God has a job for you in a field that you would never expect, and this will prepare you for the ministry." A week later, I was hired at a mental health hospital as a psychiatric care specialist working with aggressive, acute psychotic male patients.

God works in the place that
he has sent us to wait.

The work was hard, but at the same time God was preparing me for other things. The journey of God leading me to my wife and calling me to the ministry was paved with darkness and painful moments in which I was unable to see the Master's handiwork. Oswald Chambers said that God works in the place that he has sent us to wait.[6]

Over the next four years, I focused on developing my people skills, learning relationship skills from church singles groups and online dating. On May 11, 2010, I met my beautiful wife, Kristen, at a café in Royal Oak, Michigan. Our relationship was steady, and after two years of dating, I proposed to her at the café where we met. God had taken me through a journey of self-awareness and refining to bring me a wife. We married on December 7, 2012.

In 2013, after reading Michael Hyatt's best seller *Platform: Get Noticed in a Noisy World*, I browsed Hyatt's website to check out his top literary agents and decided to email the first agent on his list, Les Stobbe. After reading my email and my theological writings, Les saw my potential and took me on as a client. Les, who is one of the cofounders of Write-to-Publish, a national Christian writer's conference which has met annually for more than four decades, suggested I write a book on autism for Christian parents.

In June 2014, my mom and I attended the Write-to-Publish Conference in Wheaton, Illinois. While Les and I were eating lunch together, my mom prayed that God would help her find some writers to eat lunch with. Moments later, a woman author in the cafeteria called to my mom, "God has reserved this seat for you." Little did my mom know, she would be sitting next to Kelli, a mother of two sons with autism and a blogger who wrote a book on autism. Kelli was instrumental in helping me interview well-known Christians with children on the spectrum and learn to publish articles on autism and special needs. She also wrote an original story included in *A Parent's Guide to Autism* in the chapter "Stories That Touch the Heart."

Refined

When God wants to make an oak tree, he takes a hundred years, but he takes only two months to make a squash. It took many years for my family to see the fruit of their labor and dedication. My mom and dad never gave up, but trusted my life to God. By Christ's grace and power, my life is fruitful. As 2 Corinthians 9:8 says, "And God is able to bless you abundantly, so that in all things at all times, having all that you need, you will abound in every good work."

Psychologist Dr. Tony Attwood describes autism as having a brain that is "wired differently." This means that the things that are processed well, special interests, can become a person's expertise. In some cases, it also means that a person on the spectrum could become a leading expert in a particular area—maybe even the best in the world.[7]

Take the time to allow your child to take what they are good at and be refined. Watch for God moments and take advantage of them. You never know how God will use your child's strengths in the future.

CLOSING THOUGHTS

God's got this, and he is still in the business of creating God moments in people's lives. Consider the diamond. A diamond is simply a chunk of coal that kept at its job. Coal is a very useful natural resource, and we're all thankful it exists. But if that coal is heated to about 2,200 degrees and some pretty intense pressure is added, it transforms into a diamond. From common to uncommon. From ordinary to extraordinary. It may take time—and some heat and pressure—but God will show you the way.

PRAYER AND MEDITATION

Prayer

God, thank you for transforming my darkness into light. Weeping may last for a night but your joy comes in the morning. Please empower me to praise and worship you in the midst of my tests and pain. Bring your faithful servants to encourage me on the autism journey. Holy Spirit, speak to my heart and enable me to recognize God moments. By your grace, make me an instrument of comfort and healing for families with children with autism. Amen.

Meditation

The light shines in the darkness, and the darkness has not overcome it. (John 1:5)

When Jacob awoke from his sleep, he thought, "Surely the LORD is in this place, and I was not aware of it." (Genesis 28:16)

Chapter 18

Eternal Perspective

*From the perspective of heaven, the most miserable life on earth
will appear as one bad night in an inconvenient hotel.*

—Teresa of Avila

*Therefore we do not lose heart. Though outwardly we are wasting
away, yet inwardly we are being renewed day by day. For our
light and momentary troubles are achieving for us an eternal
glory that far outweighs them all. So we fix our eyes not on what
is seen, but on what is unseen, since what is seen is temporary,
but what is unseen is eternal.*

—2 Corinthians 4:16–18

I TRAVEL AND speak at over seventy events a year, including more than
twenty education conferences. In 2017, my wife, Kristen, and I were
traveling to South Bend, Indiana, where I would be a featured speaker
with Coach Michael Brey at the University of Notre Dame's Play Like a
Champion Today conference. To save a little money on travel expenses,
we decided to stay at a cheap hotel for only seventy dollars a night. Little
did we know what a mistake it would be! As we entered the room, we

noticed a horrible stench—rotting fish mixed with feet fungus—seeping from the restroom. Peering into the tub, I saw a towel with brown streak marks. I also noticed the cleaning staff left no shampoo or soap. The honey badger was about to make a guest appearance in South Bend. Furious, I rode the elevator back down to the service desk and blurted out, "My room has a strange fish-feet odor, and there is no shampoo!"

"Oh, I see," the receptionist responded. "We had a busy night with many people coming and going, so we weren't able to clean all the rooms. Also, we don't supply shampoo for our guests anymore, but you can purchase a small container from the vending machine for only $2.99."

To top everything off, the toilet made a squeaky rodent noise all night. As we checked out the next morning, the receptionist asked, "How was your stay?"

Holding my tongue in check, to avoid blurting out an extremely rude comment I would later regret, I smiled and simply replied, "I wouldn't keep the lights on."

It's okay to acknowledge the frustration on the parenting journey, but don't get stuck there.

I was expecting a comfortable, clean place to stay, not the Bates Motel, and my expectations weren't met. At all. But isn't life like this sometimes too? Our expectations are not always fulfilled as we desire: neat and comfortable . . . especially when we have a child on the spectrum. We desire so much for them and often struggle with what feels like life's version of the Bates Motel, and it's easy to forget that this is just a temporary stopping point. This difficult place is not our final destination.

Keeping a positive attitude and standing firm in faith are the key ingredients when hope seems out of reach (Proverbs 13:12). Faith in God and a future with hope require us to fight daily for our children and cling to the Father.

It's okay to acknowledge the frustration on the parenting journey, but don't get stuck there. Once you've expressed your feelings, dust yourself off and continue moving forward. From an eternal perspective, we can see and experience God's grace and power, even when our hope is deferred as parents because "we live by faith, not by sight" (2 Corinthians 5:7). By hope, we trust that God is present in times of pain and will bring us through to a moment of life and resurrection. Hope gives us the ability to remember how God has been present and loving in the past and believe that it is also true in the present moment and will be true in the future.

When we see the world from our limited perspective, we get stuck thinking in one dimension. We ask, "How will this affect me?" as if the world revolves around us. When something bad like a car accident happens to someone else, we think, "Thank God that didn't happen to me."

Living with an eternal perspective of hope, on the other hand, opens our eyes to see beyond the here and now. We begin to see God's beauty in creation and respond with acts of kindness and love to those in need. Spending our moments with purpose includes teaching a handicapped child to draw, comforting an elderly man who just lost his beloved wife, or enjoying the waves of the ocean and the feel of sand between your toes. All these can be eternal moments as we worship God and take delight in his wonder. These eternal moments will find fulfillment through the resurrecting power of God, into the new creation that God will bring when Christ returns. As believers, we can have hope now and hope in our future and our child's future.

To hear, firsthand, the unexpected blessings that can be found within autism and disability, I interviewed Becky Sharrock from Australia. She has an amazing mind, and her story has been featured on *Good Morning Britain*, *60 Minutes Australia*, and in a *Ripley's Believe It or Not* comic strip. She lives with an eternal perspective, enjoying life and remembering every detail of her life since she was only twelve days old.

Becky Sharrock: An Autobiographical Mind

Becky's mom, Janet, noticed her daughter was unique.[1] As a toddler, Becky screamed when cuddled. Becky shares, "I can remember every detail from my infant years. It felt unnatural to me to be held. For fun, I would organize the cutlery drawer, read atlases, and assemble jigsaw puzzles."

On her first birthday, Becky's mom gave her a Minnie Mouse doll. "I was absolutely terrified of it, yet I couldn't tell my mum that Minnie's face scared me because I was too young to speak."

At six years old, Becky was misdiagnosed with childhood depression. When Becky was fifteen, her mom examined the diagnostic criteria and characteristics for autism and decided to have Becky tested. Clinical testing confirmed her mom's intuition that Becky was autistic. Becky shares, "Since I was diagnosed at fifteen, autism has affected virtually every aspect of my life, as I have almost all of the characteristics. It's taking me longer to mature into adulthood, find a career, and live independently."

> "Those of us with autism and other disabilities require multiple times the work to get the same acknowledgment as others."

Becky's main struggle with autism is that the world is primarily structured for neurotypical people. She states, "Those of us with autism and other disabilities require multiple times the work to get the same acknowledgment as others."

Some sensory challenges Becky experiences relate to certain sounds, smells, and sights. "I am totally terrified of balloons popping. Low buzzing background sounds cause me to experience anxiety. My sensitivity to smells can cause me to visually relive past events in my mind. The smell of honeysuckle causes me to experience anxiety because a house I didn't like going to as a child had a garden full of that scent. Whenever I come across that fragrance, I remember being bullied there. I also don't like the sight of bare feet, so I wear my Converse sneakers in the house."

Despite these struggles, she has developed some helpful coping skills. "For loud sounds, I've learned to discreetly adapt by listening to music through my Bose headphones. These headphones are the best because they're soft, custom-fitted, wireless with a long-lasting battery, and able to block background noise. With scents, I'm beginning to use my sensitive nose to reproduce happy memories. I use drops of fragrant oils on a handkerchief such as peppermint to remind me of my favorite candy shops from childhood or happy holiday occasions."

Becky, from infancy, possessed an incredible memory. She is able to perfectly recall every event in her life from twelve days old; her earliest memory is lying on a sheepskin in the front seat of a car, looking up at the steering wheel and thinking, "What is this?"

"When I get a memory, I relive it vividly; I know it's not real, but my emotions think it is. I can even remember every birthday of mine." Her amazing memory applies to reading as well. Becky loves Harry Potter and can recite all seven books.

She does not have a photographic memory, but her mind has the powerful ability to recollect a sequence of events down to the microscopic details. "My short-term memory is poor, but after a month it becomes long-term, which stays forever."

If you give Becky a random day from twenty years back, she can tell you the day of the week it was, what foods she ate, the weather, her outfit, and every detail in precise order of what she saw and heard.

There are some drawbacks to her memory ability. When Becky was in elementary school, bullies noticed she was different and tormented her. "My memory ability makes it difficult to release negative memories and causes me to relive them. I also experience frequent bouts with insomnia, fatigue, and headaches from all the clutter in my mind." Whenever Becky recalls a childhood injury, she physically feels the pain again.

In fourth grade, Becky dreaded recess because it was hard to socialize and deal with bullies. A kind teacher, Mrs. Judy, lent her a copy of *Harry Potter and the Sorcerer's Stone* to read. Harry Potter helped her learn how to interpret her emotions and control her thoughts. She was able to relate with Harry Potter who felt alone and different and had magical abilities that enabled him to make friends. "Very soon I made friends of my own and dreaded recess no longer."

Becky admits that she felt rather skeptical at first about the book series, but after reading a few chapters, she connected with the book. "In a mere two weeks, I bought my own copy, and have read and reread the books continually for the past eighteen years."

From childhood to her teenage years, Becky thought her memory ability was like everyone else's. Then, on January 23, 2011, as Becky was feeding her guinea pig, her parents said, "Becky, come quickly! You need to see these people on *60 Minutes*. They have a memory ability just like yours! It's called highly superior autobiographical memory."

"What's so amazing about that?" Becky asked.

Becky's mom contacted the University of California, Irvine, and UC's research team had her travel from Australia to California. After several tests, Becky was diagnosed with HSAM and included in the UC Irvine's Stark Labs study. Only eighty people in the world have been diagnosed with HSAM, and Becky was the first from Australia.

Becky shares, "One benefit of HSAM is I have an amazing story to tell people about myself. Yet, most importantly, it gives me an opportunity to contribute to neurological research. This hopefully can lead to the prevention, or even cure, of Alzheimer's, which my grandfather had."

Becky is currently writing an autobiography called *My Life Is a Puzzle*. "In my book, I share my first memories up to the present, including my experiences with autism and HSAM, what it was like when Mum met my stepdad who had three daughters younger than me, and how we became a happy family."

Becky is also working on achieving her dreams of gaining independence. "Ever since I was diagnosed with autism and severe anxiety as a teenager, it was my dream to be able to live independently and have a career. I was told by the psychologist during my diagnosis that it was highly unlikely I would achieve any of those things. Yet I didn't lose hope. Instead, I put all of my hope in God and heaven.

"As a result of my severe anxiety, I need to be on medication, which unfortunately makes me unable to drive a car. However, I'm now being introduced to public transportation including buses, trains, and ferries. This is very scary, yet I'm praying for comfort along the way, which is helping me immensely. It's also nice and exciting that my life is opening up to a much more independent life.

"Now, at thirty years old, I'm further along than anyone back then could have imagined I'd be. My independent skills have improved enormously and brought new opportunities. Developing a speaking and writing career has greatly improved my social and communication skills. Now

I'm working on further developing these skills, connections, experiences, and qualifications to become a professor in the field of neuropsychology.

"The work involved can be quite scary. Yet now I trust that if God was able to alleviate my pain so effectively from when I was a teenager, he could help me to do anything I strongly desire, just as long as I trust and have complete faith in both him and heaven."

While the negative memories are always with her, she chooses to focus on her positive experiences and use her story and unique skills to help others. Like Becky, we also can find hope in our treasured memories and choose to focus on the eternal.

CLOSING THOUGHTS

In Colossians 3:2 the apostle Paul reminds us, "Set your minds on things above, not on earthly things." In this life we will experience times of trials—delays in development or meltdowns—but we will also experience abundance, seeing God's hand on our children's lives and the amazing people God sends along our paths to bless us. Living life from an eternal perspective and trusting God with our present and our futures will help us hold on to hope and faith.

PRAYER AND MEDITATION

Prayer

Open my eyes, God, to see life through the lens of eternity, living by faith, not sight. You're an ever-present help in time of trouble. Today I give you my anxiety and worry because you care for me. Place me in the shield of your protection—the palm of your hand. Remind me in times of distress that my hope is found in Christ and my reward is from my God. Amen.

Meditation

> Better is one day in your courts than a thousand elsewhere; I would rather be a doorkeeper in the house of my God than dwell in the tents of the wicked. (Psalm 84:10)

But our citizenship is in heaven. And we eagerly await a Savior from there, the Lord Jesus Christ, who, by the power that enables him to bring everything under his control, will transform our lowly bodies so that they will be like his glorious body. (Philippians 3:20–21)

Chapter 19

Answers to Prayers

No measure of faith is preserved without prayer.
—JEROME OF STRIDON

Before they call I will answer;
while they are still speaking I will hear.
—ISAIAH 65:24

WHEN I WAS diagnosed with autism in 1982, my mom and dad continually prayed for God's wisdom and guidance in parenting. My parents believed—and still do believe—that prayer is powerful and effective, requiring us to place our trust in Christ and wait patiently for God's provision. From an early age, my parents taught my brothers and me to pray. Every night, our family had bedtime prayers. When I experienced struggles and doubts, my dad said, "Ron, there is only one thing to do: pray and trust God."

Dad was just telling me to do what Jesus often did. He often "withdrew to lonely places and prayed" (Luke 5:16). During these times of prayer in lonely or deserted places, God empowered Jesus for ministry. Finding time for prayer can be challenging when you have a child with autism.

You likely go to bed exhausted after your child has had a meltdown or after hearing about disturbing behavioral issues from your child's school. Despite this, making time to pray is vital to finding peace. My parents taught me five valuable lessons of prayer.

1. Prayer changes our perspective but not always our circumstances.

Søren Kierkegaard writes, "Prayer does not change God, but it changes him or her who prays."[1] As a child, I often prayed for God to take away my learning disabilities or make me popular and a great athlete. I even prayed a few times for God to bring me a girlfriend—not just any girl but the prettiest blonde in the school. Of course, God does not answer every prayer like a cosmic genie. Through prayer, we learn to see things from God's perspective and hear his Holy Spirit.

God did not take away my learning disabilities but through prayer helped me receive the accommodations I needed like tutoring, note takers, and awesome proofreaders. One of my proofreaders from ORU went on to receive his PhD from Duke and became a professor.

Prayer also causes us to be more sensitive to God's presence and plans. Pastor Jason Hague shares:

> My experience isn't big enough to make conclusions about the whole of reality, or about the goodness of an omnipresent, eternal God. Just because I am going through some difficult times doesn't mean God isn't answering prayers. He might, in fact, be answering my neighbor's prayer. He might be blessing my coworkers or family members in some beautiful ways. It is essential that I open my eyes to these blessings, even if I am not the one who benefits, because they prove that God is still active and still working toward the benefit of his people. When we take time to acknowledge his work in others, it can still tempt us toward jealousy, but we don't have to go there. Rather, we can celebrate such victories as if they were our own. We can import celebration.[2]

As you pray, be careful that you don't compare your child's progress to his peers. It's okay to express those hurts, but make it your main focus to pray for wisdom and for the Holy Spirit to direct you to the right professionals and resources for your child. When I speak at churches or conferences I pray for God's connections. These people help open doors for more speaking and ministry opportunities.

2. Prayer is communication with God.

In friendships, like prayer, we sometimes ask for help in times of troubles. Psalm 50:15 says, "Call upon Me in the day of trouble; I will deliver you, and you shall glorify Me" (NKJV). After the battery on my Saturn Ion died, I asked my coworker and friend Toby to take me to an auto parts store to help me purchase a new battery. The fact that I asked Toby to assist me shows that I trusted him to deliver me safely to the store and trusted his ability to help me choose a good replacement; and his helping me, even though it was inconvenient for him, is a sign that he saw me as a friend too. Similarly, when my wife, daughter, and I had ear infections and fevers of 103.5, the only prayer I could whimper was, "God, help us!"

Prayer doesn't make things easier.
Prayer makes things possible.

Over time these little acts of request and supply build a relationship. But as Oswald Chambers writes, prayer is meant to be more than just a way of "getting things for ourselves . . . the biblical purpose of prayer is that we may get to know God Himself."[3]

If your friend only ever asked you for favors, it wouldn't be much of a friendship. It's the same with God. He desires not only for us us to offer prayers asking for provision and help but also for us to commune with him. Sharing in prayer with the Creator, we can release our fears, distress, hopes, and desires to him. As we pray, God reveals his love for us and also brings us peace and comfort.

3. We feel refreshed when we pray.

I love to go for walks in the woods and pray to God. Nature is a great environment to feel refreshed and connected with the Almighty: "For since the creation of the world God's invisible qualities—his eternal power and divine nature—have been clearly seen, being understood from what has been made" (Romans 1:20). And remember Jesus's practice of going off alone to talk to God the Father? When we engage in this healthy practice, it frees our minds of the busyness of life and enables us to hear God's voice too.

4. Answers to prayer often take time and patience.

Prayer doesn't make things easier. Prayer makes things possible. Sometimes God does instantly answer our prayers, but such a response is the exception—not the rule. Second Chronicles 29:36 records, "Hezekiah and all the people rejoiced at what God had brought about for his people, because it was done so quickly." Often we experience anxiety and discomfort as we wait for God to answer our prayers. The prophet Jonah can testify to this. He spent three long days and nights in the belly of a huge, smelly fish before his prayer for deliverance was answered (Jonah 2:1).

In middle school, I was bullied and only had one close friend. I prayed for God to help me to develop friendships. Four years later, my prayers were answered as I had friends on the track team. My parents prayed thirty-seven years for God to bring me a wife who would love me all the days of my life. They saw how depressed I was when my friends from college were getting married, and I was the lone bachelor. It took me fifteen years after college . . . and many heartbreaks . . . before finally meeting my wife.

5. God is faithful and guides our lives through prayer.

Isaiah 30:21 says, "Whether you turn to the right or to the left, your ears will hear a voice behind you, saying, 'This is the way; walk in it.'" As we pray, the Holy Spirit speaks to our hearts, revealing God's path. My parents taught me to listen to God's voice in prayer. As you pray, God will direct your steps and also bring the right therapists, specialists, and teachers to help your child with autism. Augustine of Hippo said that

God gives where he finds empty hands.[4] God is looking for open hearts and a willingness to receive what he provides.

Prayer teaches us perseverance and trust. Steve and Miranda Keskes, both educators, have been learning the humbling power of prayer while raising their ten-year-old son, Connor, who has high-functioning autism.

Connor Keskes: The Power of Praying Parents

Steve and Miranda welcomed their first son, Connor, into the world in August of 2010.[5] He was stubborn even before birth; he was born eleven days late after his mother was induced . . . on two separate occasions. It was an otherwise procedural birth, and he was a happy baby. He was baptized at three months old and began attending day care while his mother went back to work teaching. Based on their experiences as educators, both parents felt confident in their ability to raise a child.

Then, at about thirteen months, something changed.

"He was crawling along the floor and became agitated," Miranda recalls. "Then, he just started banging his head repeatedly along the hardwood. I was so scared he would hurt himself."

This moment jump-started a series of aggressive episodes. Connor physically unleashed his frustration and feelings of overstimulation, which his parents later learned was because he was sensory-seeking. He was repeatedly removed from day cares for hitting, pulling hair, scratching, and biting, all for seemingly "no reason."

"That was probably the most frustrating part," Miranda shares. "I know behavior is always a reaction to something, but I couldn't figure out what the antecedent was. I felt frustrated with myself because I didn't know how to help him. Kids were scared of him, but I could tell he desperately wanted to play with them."

His aggression was unleashed at home as well. At three years old, he would have meltdowns that resulted in his entire room being torn apart. He would throw things and hit both his mother and baby brother. Both parents were beside themselves, trying every parenting trick in the book, but none of them seemed to work.

Eventually, it was their pediatrician who advised that they see a specialist after watching him run in circles, unable to make eye contact, and touching the walls repeatedly during a well-child visit.

"I remember taking him to U of M hospital and watching him in the waiting room touch every single chair," Steve recalls. "When they diagnosed him with autism, it was sort of a relief. I had been praying that we'd find whatever we needed to help him, but at the same time, we were shocked. God had provided us with an answer, but it wasn't the one we'd been expecting."

Since Connor's diagnosis, Steve and Miranda have had the ability to support his growth through a variety of therapies and supports at school. He was able to attend two preschools concurrently: a preschool for the neurotypical, and a preschool for children with diverse needs. He has an IEP at school, ensuring he gets the sensory breaks he needs and frequent practice interacting with others. He also attends social skills groups, both in school and privately.

At six years old, Connor came to the realization on his own that he was "different." In tears, he revealed to his mother that he "felt like a robot" and was "scared of the thoughts in his head." Soon after, his parents introduced him to a child psychologist who shared with Connor his diagnosis.

Miranda shares, "When Connor was told he had autism, he asked me, 'Why did God make me this way?' With sincerity, I told him God had big plans for him. To me, that was the beginning of his faith journey. It's been rocky at times—he loves to question everything, which I love about him—but the desire to believe in God is there. All we can continue to do is foster it through prayer."

His father shares, "I am a firm believer that God doesn't give you everything you want; God gives you what you need. That's something to be mindful of. God answers prayers on his timeline, not our timeline."

Trusting in God's timeline, Steve and Miranda continue to model patience, teaching Connor the gift of prayer as well. It's often a struggle for him. Steve explains, "Faith is intangible and requires patience, but Connor wants instant gratification. Connor trusts things he can see and feel, because to him that's the only way."

When Connor can find God in concrete ways, his faith seems to grow. He takes pride in wearing the gold cross he received for his First Communion, and he spends hours reading his Bible graphic novel.

Steve shares, "Our faith has helped Connor work through sensory challenges as well. For Ash Wednesday, it's customary to put ashes on your forehead. Connor has a strong aversion to any sort of face paint, so putting ash on his forehead was really uncomfortable for him. The ashes themselves are an abstract concept as well. It tested him both physically and intellectually.

"Something you have to understand about Connor is that he doesn't believe anything interacts outside of the brain. Connor is very cerebral." Steve continues, "When I think about my soul, I can feel every hair in my body stand up. I feel a fuzziness in my fingertips and toes. It's a sensory experience for me. But for Connor, because he is sensory-seeking, it seems to be harder for him to connect with that."

Helping Connor have faith in God is essential to Steve. "Both of my parents came from very meager upbringings. It was constantly said in my house, 'If you have nothing else in this world, you have your education, and you have your faith.' Those two things will help you get through this world and the next."

Steve and Miranda continue to instill these values in their own boys. "Life is full of challenge. It's not easy." Steve explains, "Connor is going to make mistakes, and he's incredibly hard on himself. I want him to have a foundation outside of himself where he can find inner peace. Divine intervention is so central to everything that we have. I continue to pray to God to reveal himself to Connor in ways he can grasp."

Steve and Miranda's prayers continue to be answered through Connor's many accomplishments. Miranda says, "Connor now has the ability to find, make, and sustain friends. He has to navigate them with a little more intention and focus than others, but he's beginning to see how his behavior impacts others. He used to think it was never his fault."

Connor has also participated and found success in soccer, wrestling, and flag football. He continues to seek out new interests, such as rock climbing and fishing. He excels academically, especially in reading and math. He's learned coping mechanisms to calm himself down, such as going into his room and reading a book. He knows it's okay to tell the adults in his life, "I need a break," and then find a quiet space.

"In first grade, his case coordinator at school figured out doing math problems is soothing for Connor," Miranda shares. "So whenever Connor was starting to feel stressed, he would simply go to a quiet place and work on math problems." She laughs. "I'm not sure many people would find multiplication soothing, but Connor certainly does!"

> "We've come to realize that it's not apathy many people with autism feel, but overwhelming emotions that cause them to shut down."

"What I'm most proud of, though," his mother continues, "is his genuine empathy for others. I was told when he was first diagnosed that he didn't have empathy because of his autism. That always made me upset because I knew, deep down, it was wrong." She shakes her head. "It shows you how far our understanding of autism has already come. Now we've come to realize that it's not apathy many people with autism feel, but overwhelming emotions that cause them to shut down.

"My prayers have always revolved around Connor forming meaningful relationships. Over time, he's been able to bend his rigid thinking and feel compassion and understanding for others, especially for his younger brother, Cameron. In so many ways, Cameron has been a gift from God, not only for us but for Connor. Cameron is naturally empathetic, and his patience with his brother is inspiring. In turn, Connor loves his brother fiercely. Their bond is something I frequently say a prayer of thanks for."

Steve explains his relationship with prayer. "Prayer is calming to me. It helps me to be humble. As a parent, I often feel we'll take five steps forward with Connor and then we get smacked in the face with a terrible interaction at school and take ten steps back. After moments like this, I pray: 'God, please help me and give me serenity.' Afterward, I always feel more at peace."

As Steve and Miranda look to the future, they reflect on their faith journey. "A connection with God is a leap of faith, a step off of a cliff. Faith is difficult. It pushes all of us," Steve shares. "I have faith that God has a wonderful plan, not only for Connor but for all of us."

"Connor's honesty is one of my favorite traits about him," his mom shares. "I asked him recently if he believed in God or not. He was quiet for a moment, then he said, 'I can't tell you if I believe in God or not. I'm still deciding. I'm young and have a lot to learn.'

"The next day, we all sat down to dinner, and Connor led the prayer."

CLOSING THOUGHTS

Connor's journey with autism has been filled with challenges, but his parents chose not to quit and, instead, continue to pray. They are now seeing the fruits of their labor through God's grace. Prayer is powerful and effective. As you continue to guide your child with autism, remember to pray and seek God. Exodus 14:14 says, "The LORD will fight for you; you need only to be still."

PRAYER AND MEDITATION

Prayer

Thank you, Father, for my child and our family. I pray that you will give me wisdom in making decisions for my child. I ask that you would reveal yourself very clearly to my child, and that they would come to have a personal relationship with you. And when I forget to speak to you, please still speak to me and remind me of your presence and loving direction for our family. Amen.

Meditation

Hear my cry for help, my King and my God, for to you I pray. In the morning, LORD, you hear my voice; in the morning I lay my requests before you and wait expectantly. (Psalm 5:2–3)

I will give thanks to you, LORD, with all my heart; I will tell of all your wonderful deeds. (Psalm 9:1)

Chapter 20

Ain't No Stoppin' Us Now

Expect great things from God; attempt great things for God.

—William Carey

Finally, be strong in the Lord and in his mighty power.

—Ephesians 6:10

My pup, Rudy, a Jack Russell terrier and Pomeranian mix, is high energy, persistent, and unstoppable. He has a go-getter temperament and the personality of the Energizer Bunny intoxicated on Red Bull. This breed loves being fully involved with the family and playing . . . hard! If you don't give them enough exercise and companionship, you're going to have a destructive pup on your hands. Some terriers are so brash that they will go toe-to-toe with a much larger and fiercer dog, given the right, or should I say wrong, mood. A honey badger trait—I love it!

Unfortunately Rudy loves to munch on Makayla's plastic toy fruits and Barbie dolls. If Kristen and I give attention to our cat, Frishma, Rudy is quick to have a canine barking meltdown. The only way to slow him down is a fast-paced two-mile run, even when Michigan is covered in ice and snow. Parents who have a child with autism and feel defeated and depressed would love to possess the energetic and determined attitude of Rudy. Colossians 1:29 says, "To this end I strenuously contend with all the energy Christ so powerfully works in me."

> The secret to continue walking forward
> on the autism journey is to find
> relentless faith in a powerful God.

There's no doubt that life with a child with autism can sap a parent of energy. But the secret to continue walking forward on the autism journey is to find relentless faith in a powerful God. My parents learned four ways to keep moving when my autism wore them down.

1. Don't allow depression to steal your family's joy.

Depression is a pervasive sadness that pulls you down. It is a very common issue for both children on the spectrum and their parents. My parents have suffered seasons of depression. It can negatively affect your work performance, health, and friendships, making it important to address.

Patrick Marlborough, a journalist and comedian, blogs:

> A depressive hibernation is not so much a purposeful exile, as a slow-paced locking of doors. When your mind feels groggy and your day is a looping cycle of inaction and despairing thoughts, it can be hard to work up the strength to go to a friend's gig, grab a coffee, or reply to a text. In my own experience, the disease does so much to convince you of your awfulness, that you start viewing your absence from friends and events as a deformed favor. You mute yourself for fear that your internal wailing will wreck the vibe for others.[1]

Depression is a thief. It'll rob you of your time, your thoughts, and your sense of self. The end results of depression are isolation and unproductivity, even death. My parents handle their depression by using a combination of medication and counseling from professional psychologists and pastors. If you're struggling, it's good to seek the advice and wisdom of others (Proverbs 24:6).

2. Accept life as it comes to you.

One of the roots of depression is feeling overwhelmed by life. My Grandpa Olmsted, who lived to be almost ninety, had a great life philosophy: "It is what it is! Don't be depressed by the future, but take life as it comes to you."

Accepting life as it comes requires flexibility and adjusting to change. You take your son to the zoo and he experiences a meltdown. Change in plan. My mom experienced many of these moments as she was raising me. She expected things in life to go wrong sometimes, and learned to always have a plan B for any situation . . . and not freak out.

I also have learned to accept life as it comes. Working in the mental health field with easily agitated psych patients can be unpredictable and dangerous. Often you have to work on a unit with new patients and different nursing staff. Being able to adjust is essential. I adjust by being confident God will protect me and adapting to my coworkers' personalities. I also pray each morning, "God, give me job security and keep me safe."

3. Receive strength and stability from God.

Depression does not always go away—my parents and I have battled it our whole lives. We can testify that God will give you strength to endure the battles but not always make the pain cease. Sometimes you, like my parents, may need to seek professional help.

Faith can empower you to deal with depression. The apostle Paul, while he was in prison, wrote, "I can endure all things through Christ who strengthens me" (Philippians 4:13, author's translation). Due to depression from severe bullying and low self-esteem, I began to drink and use drugs my freshman year of high school. I quit attending youth group activities and began to make unwise choices in friends.

By the beginning of my junior year, I was smoking marijuana daily and drinking almost every weekend. I felt hopeless inside and had no motivation for academics or athletics. My GPA was only 1.7 during those two and a half years of darkness.

The middle of my junior year of high school, a senior who attended both my school and my church said, "We miss seeing you at our youth group. God's doing awesome things. You should come next Wednesday night and be a part!" That Wednesday night, I attended youth group and the message spoke to my heart. I rededicated my life to following Christ. Over the next month, I quit drinking, drugs, tobacco, and even swearing. I made new friends in the youth group and became focused again on sports, education, and Christ.

God's grace and love transformed my life. The Holy Spirit spoke to my heart to memorize the Bible. By memorizing the Scriptures, God empowered me to make the honor roll and graduate with a 2.5 GPA. Through the Word of God, my life became more stable, and the depression more bearable.

4. Live a life of worship.

Worship paves a powerful path leading from melancholy to joy. King David proclaimed, "I will sing the LORD's praise, for he has been good to me" (Psalm 13:6). I love to sing worship songs to God like "How Great Is Our God" by Chris Tomlin or "Awesome God" by Rich Mullins.[2] These classic worship songs fill my heart with joy and encourage me to trust God in the midst of my depression. Psalm 42:8 says, "By day the LORD directs his love, at night his song is with me—a prayer to the God of my life." One of my favorite energizing verses on worship is Psalm 40:3: "He put a new song in my mouth, a hymn of praise to our God. Many will see and fear the LORD and put their trust in him."

Worship helps create an unstoppable faith that will carry us through life's difficult times.

But worship isn't just praise music. A quick look at Scripture tells us that being grateful, admiring nature, and listening to or reading the Bible are all forms of worship, as is doing what we're called to do and working to the best of our abilities (Psalms 103:2; 104).

When we take time to worship, it takes the focus off our seemingly impossible situation and puts it on God, who is "able to do immeasurably more than all we ask or imagine" (Ephesians 3:20). In combination with listening to the wise advisors God puts in our lives, worship helps create an unstoppable faith that will carry us through life's difficult times. Tarik El-Abour demonstrates the power of an unstoppable faith with his passion for baseball and his ability to overcome every challenge.

Tarik El-Abour: The First Professional Baseball Player with Autism

Nadia Khalil had a two-year-old daughter, so she knew her son Tarik's milestones were delayed.[3] Tarik, unlike his older sister, did not make eye contact or respond to her voice. He experienced ticks from Tourette's syndrome, and he lined up his toy cars and trains in perfect rows. He would not interact with other children, and he hated loud noises. He was a great observer, watching others rather than wanting to socialize with them.

Nadia shares, "We had a birthday party for our daughter with Barney and friends. Tarik loved the characters in *Barney & Friends*, yet when he saw the purple dinosaur, he ran in terror from our home. I started immediately to search for answers to try to learn how his mind processed information.

"When Tarik was nonverbal, I checked his comprehension to understand commands and hearing ability by placing three cars on the floor—red, blue, and yellow cars. 'Pick up the yellow one,' I told him. Tarik proceeded to pick up the yellow car. This made me know he could understand and hear me."

A few months before Tarik was diagnosed with autism, Nadia had a vivid dream of Tarik jumping in a pool with no water while she screamed, "Help him! He does not understand!" Nadia struggled immensely with what to do.

After intensive testing, Tarik was diagnosed with autism at age three.

"I was determined to bridge the gap between my world and Tarik's so I could help him learn new skills. Early on, I taught Tarik that not everything is one way or the other but we can make choices in life. I did this by placing three or four toys before him and saying, 'What toy do you want to play with today?' He learned best through rote learning. Tarik thinks in numbers. If it worked twice, it should work a third time also. One step at a time. I made a decision not to medicate him. I went back to school and took classes at UCLA through their extension program and studied childhood development."

Tarik was nonverbal until age six. When Tarik first began to speak, he hit his leg each time he tried to pronounce a word and Nadia replied, "Let's try it again." Tarik was a very picky eater and only ate five foods: cookies, doughnuts, pizza, spaghetti, and hamburgers. Nadia encouraged him to try new foods by not making a separate meal for him and stating, "This new recipe is delicious. Please try it, and let me know what you think."

Tarik learned he had autism his final year of middle school. "I just addressed the symptoms of autism. As Tarik matured, I did not have a formal conversation to inform him he was on the spectrum. However, I did have conversations with his school on how to bring out Tarik's best. I treated him as any other child because I noticed he emulates. I was *very* careful about what I exposed him to so he could shoot higher and higher."

Nadia's unstoppable faith in Christ empowered her in raising Tarik. "God has been our rock. Our source of strength—the grace to face all the challenges with autism and overcoming them. Through Christ's love and compassion, our family is able to share God's love and encourage others facing autism."

When Tarik was seven, Nadia was walking across the street and got hit by a car. Later that day, due to a concussion, she was unable to recall her children's names. After this crisis, Nadia thought, "What if I would've died? Who would take care of my children? I must teach them to be independent and advocate for themselves."

Tarik's greatest challenge to overcome was his lack of social skills. Nadia shares, "Social skills were difficult for Tarik and still are. Reading others, feeling understood, socializing, and trying new things take him longer to learn and assimilate."

When Tarik was ten years old, his father took him to a local baseball tryout. He was the worst player on the field since he had never played baseball and didn't understand the rules of the game. Despite his lack of playing skills, Tarik fell in love with baseball. The excitement of watching the players, the colorful outfits, the bright lights, and the roar of the crowd sparked his interest. "What drove him was his love for the game. He would do anything to play baseball. Tarik loved everything about baseball from the smell of the grass in the field to standing at the plate. That day he discovered his passion in life."

Nadia encouraged Tarik's passion. "I followed his love. I gave him all the opportunities and was his biggest fan. I loved going to the games and helping Tarik find new teams to play for. He played baseball constantly and loved to imitate his favorite player, Jackie Robinson, sliding in to home plate."

When Tarik was twelve and playing little league, Nadia picked him up after a game. As he entered the car, he was frustrated and stated, "I wished I could've hit a home run today."

"Tarik, you've never hit a home run, so why are you upset about it today?"

"I wanted to hit one today," Tarik replied.

"You know, if you hit a ground ball, someone is liable to mess up and then you can get on base," Nadia explained.

"Mom, I do not want to be a success on someone else's mistake. I want to be successful because I am successful."

Tarik's teammates couldn't understand his passion. He was the first on the field and the last to leave. While his teammates were enjoying social events, Tarik was busy taking extra batting practice or fielding fly balls in the outfield.

"Being autistic, this was completely normal to Tarik. His briefcase was his baseball bag. He found friends to play catch. He even paid a few pitchers to throw so he could practice batting. He would run sprints around the ballpark, engage in plyometric exercises, and began eating healthy. The key to Tarik's eventual success on the field is his work ethic," Nadia reveals.

Tarik's hard work on the field, integrity, and relentless pursuit of the game caused his high school baseball coach, a former college player and pro, to mentor him and help him develop the skills to reach the next level.

Tarik's goal in life was to play professional ball. Nadia shares, "He told me that when he grew up and played baseball, he would buy me a house wherever he plays, so I could watch his games live. He did not know yet how different he was. He did not know yet how autism was going to speak for him before he could speak for himself."

After graduating from San Marino High School, he played baseball briefly at Pasadena City College. As a sophomore, Tarik was redshirted. Tarik was heartbroken and depressed; however, his junior year he played as an outfielder and provided key hits. When Tarik was redshirted, he continued to play ball with his teammates and improve his skills while waiting for his next opportunity.

The next year, he received a $5,000 scholarship to play baseball at Concordia University in California, but he was cut two weeks before the season began. With tears in his eyes, he told his mom, "We need to find a team where I can play ball." He transferred to Pacifica College and played a year there, and the next year, the school merged with Bristol University.

After graduating from Bristol University with a Bachelor of Science in business administration, Tarik signed with the independent Empire League and played for the Sullivan Explorers in southern New York. He hit .323 and won rookie of the year honors. In 2017, he hit .240 for the Plattsburgh Red Birds, helping them win the championship.

Tarik and his parents refused to give up and pushed through difficult circumstances, accepting life as it came, but also receiving strength and stability from God. And a domino effect began to occur. Tarik's former high school mentor contacted Reggie Sanders, who works for the Kansas City Royals. Sanders is a former major league baseball player and has a forty-year-old brother with autism.

A longtime advocate for those on the spectrum, Sanders approached the Royals about letting Tarik take batting practice prior to a game. They agreed. It was easy to see that Tarik was a natural fit. Some months later, Sanders approached the general manager about offering Tarik a minor league contract.

"The repetitiveness of autism and the repetitiveness of baseball go hand in hand. Tarik can be an asset to our organization by providing passion and love for the game, as well as his skills," Sanders said.

The Royals organization has a history of promoting inclusion of neurodivergent individuals. Also, Reggie Sanders founded RSFCares, a network of support for children and families living with autism.[4] When Tarik received the news from his mom that the Royals were signing him to a minor league deal, he ran around the house, repeating, "I can't believe this—all I ever wanted was to play baseball!" After his first extended spring training game, Tarik called Sanders to say, "I'm in the right place."

Nadia states, "There is nowhere else in this world I'd rather be than with my children." She encourages parents who have a child with autism, "Don't compromise your child's confidence or learning ability. The more confidence you have in them, the more they will have in themselves. Have faith God will provide a way and guide you."

Depression from being cut from baseball teams did not keep Tarik from playing professional ball. Instead, Tarik was unstoppable in his pursuit to accomplish his dream.

CLOSING THOUGHTS

Nadia refused to allow autism to limit Tarik's pursuit of playing baseball. She encouraged Tarik to follow his dreams and use the gifts God gave him. When Tarik felt depressed from not making a team or being cut, his mom encouraged him to keep pursuing his dreams. An unstoppable faith that helps us deal with depression requires us to accept life as it comes, worship God for his goodness, rely on Christ's strength, and not allow depression to steal our joy. As the apostle Paul stated, "Be joyful in hope, patient in affliction, faithful in prayer" (Romans 12:12).

PRAYER AND MEDITATION

Prayer

God, I need you to provide food and water in this emotional desert. Transform the burning sand into pools of grace, the thirsty ground into bubbling springs of abundance. Refresh my weary soul and empower me to press forward to the high calling in Christ Jesus. Let my faith in you be relentless and unstoppable. Bless my family and place them in the protective shadow of your wings. Amen.

Meditation

> I press on, that I may lay hold of that for which Christ Jesus has also laid hold of me. (Philippians 3:12 NKJV)

> One thing I do: Forgetting what is behind and straining toward what is ahead, I press on toward the goal to win the prize for which God has called me heavenward in Christ Jesus. (Philippians 3:13–14)

Chapter 21

The Race Marked Out for Us

Tell me I can't so I can show you that I can.
—ARMANI WILLIAMS, NASCAR DRIVER DIAGNOSED WITH AUTISM

*However, I consider my life worth nothing to me; my only aim is
to finish the race and complete the task the Lord Jesus has given
me—the task of testifying to the good news of God's grace.*
—ACTS 20:24

ANY FOOL CAN see an apple on a tree, but it takes vision and dedication
to see apple orchards in the seeds. My mom never allowed teachers' or
doctors' professional opinions to limit my potential. She believed Jesus's
promise in Matthew 19:26, "With man this is impossible, but with God
all things are possible." My mom fixed her eyes on Jesus and trusted my
care into the Father's hands, believing God would use my autism and
disabilities for his glory. She also prayed God would bring the right therapists and teachers to work with me. But she also never expected this apple
seed to turn into an orange. She never asked me to be something I wasn't.
She simply asked me to be the best I could be, and she never wavered
from that.

As the author of the book of Hebrews says, "Let us run with perseverance the race marked out for us, fixing our eyes on Jesus, the pioneer and perfecter of faith. For the joy set before him he endured the cross, scorning its shame, and sat down at the right hand of the throne of God. Consider him who endured such opposition from sinners, so that you will not grow weary and lose heart" (Hebrews 12:1–3).

Each one of us has our own race marked out for us, a unique and specific path that God has laid out. I have found five ways to run the race.

1. Never lose heart—just keep getting up.

My mom refused to lose heart. She knew by experience that autism, "the race marked out for our family," was not a sprint, but a marathon. Every milestone and big event in my life took me longer than my peers and brothers: I graduated from high school at twenty, I was thirty-five years old before I had a long-term relationship, thirty-six when I moved out of my parents' home, thirty-seven when I got married, forty-one when I became a father, forty-two when my first book was published, and forty-three for my second book, *Thought, Choice, Action: Decision-Making That Releases the Holy Spirit's Power.*

Deborah Reber, whose son Asher has Asperger's, writes: "I'm convinced that the greatest gift we can give our differently wired kids is the knowledge of who they are, how their brain works, and what they need to do to create the life they want. Because when we guide our children along the path of self-discovery, they can feel good about themselves, develop self-advocacy skills, and ultimately grow up to be self-realized adults."[1]

2. Be prepared by understanding your child's needs.

My mom studied my behavioral patterns to understand the situations leading to my meltdowns. From ages three to six, my meltdowns were caused mainly by touch, sounds, and smells. If a stranger touched my arm or patted my back, I would experience a meltdown; the smell of nail polish or salmon would bring the honey badger out of his burrow.

At age eight, while on vacation out west, I saw the nastiest pair of feet—this lady's toenails were yellowish brown and shaped and textured like campanelle noodles. After this, for the next three years, the sight of bare feet gave me an instant meltdown. My dad helped me overcome this phobia by taking me to the beach and rewarding me with a red, white, and blue popsicle for handling the sight of bare feet.

Don't let obstacles slow you down for long; take a deep breath, make an alternate plan, and get moving again.

Understanding my own daughter's needs has become easier as she has gained language. Recently, she pointed out the window while I was writing and said, "Daddy, look! Colorful leaves! Let's collect them." Recognizing her need for playtime, we spent the afternoon collecting and creating artwork from the leaves.

Julie Hornok, whose teenage daughter Lizzie has autism, describes the marathon mindset: "Love your child exactly as she is. We often think we need to 'fix' our children with autism, but in actuality we need to learn how their minds work and use their strengths to help them become the best version of themselves. Also, keep a marathon mindset. As parents, we want to do everything possible to help our kids, but we ourselves burn out. When we forget to take care of ourselves, our kids can feel our stress. Slow down and remember the little steps of progress will add up."[2]

3. Learn from your setbacks.

Every person reading this book will have setbacks in life, regardless of whether you have autism or not. We will all encounter obstacles as we pursue goals. In many cases, however, we can anticipate what could block our path and be prepared to move around them. Don't let obstacles slow you down for long; take a deep breath, make an alternate plan, and get moving again.

When preparing my IEPs, my mom anticipated the areas I would need extra help, like reading comprehension and spelling. She made sure those skills were included in the IEP. When my family experienced setbacks, like me repeating kindergarten, my mom encouraged me to make new friends by having fun days at home with pizza, pop, and video games.

4. Do good deeds.

The apostle Paul wrote, "Therefore, as we have opportunity, let us do good to all people" (Galatians 6:10). It's a command to do good things, so we should do it. But one thing I've learned is that God's commands are often for our own benefit. Does it help others when we help them? Of course. But science has proven that if we make time to help others, we also fuel our own hearts, reduce stress, and avoid depression.[3]

Raising a child with autism can be depressing, isolating, and draining, but we don't have to do it on our own. Second Corinthians 8:1–3 describes God's grace that empowers us to accomplish good deeds: "And now, brothers and sisters, we want you to know about the grace that God has given the Macedonian churches. In the midst of a very severe trial, their overflowing joy and their extreme poverty welled up in rich generosity. For I testify that they gave as much as they were able, and even beyond their ability." Do you see it? The Macedonians, while in extreme poverty, "welled up in rich generosity" through the grace God gave them. It should be our goal to do the same.

5. Run with confidence and faith.

God is faithful and will equip you for the race by supplying your needs "according to the riches of his glory in Christ Jesus" (Philippians 4:19).

> Even with divine favor, things don't
> always go as we planned.

We have confidence since God's favor is upon our lives. We feel his favor when we choose the right therapists or programs, or when our child has teachers who are able to relate to him and refine his gifts. Psalm 90:17 says, "May the favor of the Lord our God rest on us; establish the work of our hands for us—yes, establish the work of our hands." But even with divine favor, things don't always go as we planned and our child's therapist may not be a good match.

Devon Still, a former NFL player and author of *Still in the Game*, writes, "Faith in God doesn't make the struggle go away. The obstacles in life don't magically disappear because you pray. But the fear of those struggles? The terror of believing that each new obstacle is somehow gonna be the end of you? *That* goes away. *That* makes you stronger. And *that* is powerful."[4]

Armani Williams: NASCAR's First Driver with Autism

Armani Williams, from Grosse Point, Michigan, is the first NASCAR driver diagnosed with autism.[5] He was nonverbal until age three—his delayed speech and lack of social interaction caused him to be diagnosed with autism at age two.

Armani shares, "My greatest challenge with having autism is the communication and social interaction. All my life I have been dealing with issues, but I have managed to steadily improve those tactics, being a little more proactive around other people, and that's going to help me in the long run as I continue to live my life with autism."

Armani's family helped him develop social skills by teaching him to start conversations and make friends. Armani says, "So once it got to the point where I was comfortable being around other people, that's when the next step came to learn how to talk and interact with people. My parents have been helping me a lot, teaching me the basics of having a conversation with someone, how to stay connected with them, how to meet people I have not met before. My parents have been very supportive of me and without their help, I don't know how my life would be today."

At age eight, the breakthrough occurred when Armani discovered his passion for racing go-karts. After finishing his first lap, Armani exclaimed, "Dad, I understand." At this moment, Armani's family recognized he had a gift from God to drive—this talent would help him to develop other skills.

Armani's love for racing thrived as he began collecting NASCAR Hot Wheels and watching all the races with his dad. "My interest in NASCAR driving started really young for me. I loved playing with my action figure cars as a kid. I would watch NASCAR nonstop, and it amazed me how fast those cars were going, passing cars, and a winner getting a trophy at the end of the race. I found that pretty cool and awesome and one day I told my dad straight up that was something I wanted to do in life: be a professional race car driver."

Armani's favorite childhood memories were of going to the racetrack with his dad. "My favorite memory was when I was ten years old and I went with my dad to my first NASCAR race: the Brickyard 400 at the Indianapolis Motor Speedway. I can remember sitting in the grandstands and seeing the racetrack, the race cars, and the racing fans with my own eyes. I had a blast, and I enjoyed the race."

Armani took advantage of every opportunity for racing. After attending a two-month camp learning the intricacies of racing the karts and subsequently winning races, he began driving racers designed for drivers as young as eight years old. Armani's triumphs in Michigan and Indiana eventually led him to the next stage of his racing career, the ARCA Truck Series, which is a pickup truck racing series that runs on tracks throughout the Midwest.

This led to a transition to stock cars in 2017, and that brought him closer to his ultimate goal of racing in the Monster Energy NASCAR Cup Series.

Armani understands the unique honor he has in racing. He's in a business that isn't always easy to break into, but he keeps getting deals put together so he can race. His goal is to learn as much as he can from every race, so he can continue his self-improvement.

Armani's on-track mentor is D. J. Kennington, the 2010 Pinty's Series champion. Kennington has been helpful to show Armani what to do—and what not to do—in the world of racing.

Since he was young, Armani has faced challenges with autism and sensory issues. "I still do today, but I have been able to reduce those issues and overcome them. When I hear or see something that I don't quite understand, I use the internet and research things on Google to help me understand. The more I learn about different things, the easier it is for me to translate the information to my brain the next time it comes up.

It's like, 'Oh, I have heard about this before,' or 'Hey, I know what this is and how to handle it.'" But autism has also given Armani an edge on the racetrack. "I find autism is an advantage for me because I'm so focused behind the wheel. That helps with being consistent, smooth, and seeing the big picture leading up to the race. It has really helped me develop as a pro race car driver."

Racing at a high level has given Armani more strengths and self-esteem and empowered him to graduate from high school with a 3.0 GPA. Armani's favorite subject? Math, because it helped him learn to problem solve and calculate numbers.

Armani finds racing to be the perfect fit. "I love to go fast and I love the competition. I love the joy of being on the racetrack and going out there and competing for wins every time I strap into a race car. Just being around the racing environment is also what I love about it, where I get to meet certain drivers, team owners, racing officials, and even talk to potential sponsors." Armani has found community.

Young adults with autism and Asperger's often struggle to learn how to drive and stay focused on the road. Armani offers these practical tips: "I tell them not to be afraid of learning something they haven't done before. Once you put in the hard work and commitment to learning the basics of working the steering wheel, the gas, and brake pedal, it will become easier and you can be more comfortable on the road, freeways, or even on the racetrack, if you want to be a race car driver."

Armani Williams encourages individuals with autism and disabilities, "If you have a dream of doing something you love, go for it. Don't give up on your dream. Stay encouraged, believe in yourself, and work hard to do what you love to do."[6]

CLOSING THOUGHTS

God will empower you with his strength and endurance to finish the race. Psalm 55:22 says, "Cast your cares on the LORD and he will sustain you; he will never let the righteous be shaken." The Scriptures promise us that we will experience trials in life, but these times of shaking will not destroy our faith, and God will reward our faithfulness. As 2 Timothy 4:7–8 says,

"I have fought the good fight, I have finished the race, I have kept the faith. Now there is in store for me the crown of righteousness, which the Lord, the righteous Judge, will award to me on that day—and not only to me, but also to all who have longed for his appearing."

PRAYER AND MEDITATION

Prayer

Father, empower me with your love and grace to run the race marked out for me. Fix my eyes on your Son, Jesus, the author and finisher of my faith. Don't let me run aimlessly, lose heart, or depart from your path. Shine your light on me. Give me vision to see the progress in my child with autism and the fruit of the Spirit you are producing in my life. Give me strength to fight the good fight and finish the race. Not by my power or might but by your Spirit. Amen.

Meditation

> Don't you realize that in a race everyone runs, but only one person gets the prize? So run to win! All athletes are disciplined in their training. They do it to win a prize that will fade away, but we do it for an eternal prize. So I run with purpose in every step. I am not just shadowboxing. I discipline my body like an athlete, training it to do what it should. (1 Corinthians 9:24–27 NLT)

> Overwhelming victory is ours through Christ, who loved us. (Romans 8:37 NLT)

Conclusion

I know of nobody who is purely autistic or
purely neurotypical. Even God had some autistic moments,
which is why the planets all spin.

—Jerry Newport, *Your Life Is Not a Label*

Now to him who is able to do immeasurably more than all we
ask or imagine, according to his power that is at work within us.

—Ephesians 3:20

At the beginning of this book, I mentioned eight characteristics of strong parents:

1. They recognize the issues to be tackled.
2. They focus on their child's strengths and abilities.
3. They celebrate their child's progress.
4. They keep a positive attitude.
5. They are fierce advocates for their child.
6. They learn to see the world from their child's perspective.
7. They never give up on their child.
8. They believe that God has a special plan for their child.

My mom, Janet, also had these eight essential qualities. This empowered me to become a husband, dad, author, international speaker, and professor. Our greatest gift for parenting is the Holy Spirit, who speaks to us and gives us God's wisdom and guidance.

Dani Bowman, an animation film producer, shares, "English is my second language. Autism is my first."[1] I am not cured of autism, but my autism is refined into beautiful talents. Your child's autism can also be refined, enabling him or her to gain independence and employment.

As Judith Newman, author of *To Siri with Love*, writes, "People with ASD don't develop skills in the kind of steady progression of neurotypical children; there's more of a herky-jerky quality to mental and emotional growth, meaning that they may not be able to do something for a very long time and then, one day, they just *can*."[2]

I call this the jack-in-the-box developmental effect; you keep trying new things, nothing seems to be working, then suddenly *pop* goes your breakthrough.

Haley Moss, the first attorney from Florida diagnosed with autism, says, "I am a work in progress. I am getting to my goal a little at a time, not all at once."[3] That's how my life has been with autism also.

> ## I am a work in progress; I still experience my autistic moments and honey badger meltdowns.

I am a work in progress; I still experience my autistic moments and honey badger meltdowns, though they are less intense and less frequent. In my parents' home, there is now an unspoken rule: "Never move or touch anything in Ron's former bedroom—it's No Man's Valley—off-limits."

My man cave houses a massive toy and book collection. Not long ago, my mom decided to move some of my toys. When I entered my man cave and saw my stuffed animals and books were out of place, my arms began to twitch like an electrical cord in water, and my hands started hitting my head. "Why, why, why did you have to move my stuff? You've ruined my collection! It's undefinable and unpredictable!" I kept screaming at the top of my lungs as I continued to lose control.

Makayla came running into the room. "Daddy, stay calm. It's okay. Sometimes McDonald's forgets to put a toy in my Happy Meal; there's always tomorrow for Grandma to get you a Happy Meal with a new toy." Makayla's gentle voice and wisdom instantly relieved me of my meltdown as I wiped the tears from my face and hugged her.

I am still learning to break free from my rigid patterns in life. I love the saying, "Those God uses the most are the ones who hold on to the least." While I was busy carrying out two boxes of books from my man cave for a speaking engagement, Makayla grabbed the unopened box of a Calico Critters Boutique set.

"Daddy, look at the beautiful purses, the cute white cat with all her jewelry, and the little shop. Can I please have this toy from your collection?" Opening the box for Makayla, I quickly learned an important lesson: nothing can break an autism routine like a beautiful four-year-old daughter.

A question I asked everyone I interviewed for this book was, "What is God teaching you?" To answer my own question, God is teaching me to trust him and release my fear and abandonment issues. As Psalm 56:3 says, "When I am afraid, I put my trust in you."

Remember to listen and learn from your children; look at their view from the spectrum.

For example, finances have always been a worry for me. Not long after I finished writing this book, we found ourselves in credit card debt due to medical expenses, groceries, and clothes for Makayla. I became afraid and experienced an anxiety attack. "Help us, God," I prayed.

The next morning, during a worship service, the Holy Spirit spoke to me and said, "Don't be afraid; trust me." After I finished speaking on "My Amazing Journey of Autism and Faith," an elder from the church handed me a check that helped pay off the bills. This has taught me that if I continue to put my trust in God, he will provide.

As you continue along the journey, remember to listen and learn from your children; look at their view from the spectrum. God is speaking through them, teaching you valuable lessons. Makayla once handed her five-year-old friend a framed picture of Grandpa Boswell and exclaimed, "I miss Grandpa Boswell; he is with Jesus." The Holy Spirit was teaching me the importance of teaching our children about Jesus and his unconditional love for us. As Proverbs 22:6 says, "Train up a child in the way he should go, and when he is old he will not depart from it" (NKJV).

Makayla's favorite request of me is, "Daddy, I want to play kitchen. You can be the chef, and Rudy and Frishma can be the customers." This is a reminder to take time off from writing and enjoy Makayla's company. Or "Let's jump on the bed!" (Disclaimer: I like doing this at hotels too and have broken my fair share.) In moments like these, the Holy Spirit reminds me to enjoy life and stay young in spirit.

I want to encourage you to never give up. Keep praying, trying new things, and reading books. Surround yourself with friends and relatives who have faith, hope, and love. As 1 Corinthians 13:13 says, "And now these three remain: faith, hope and love. But the greatest of these is love."

Acknowledgments

VIEWS FROM THE *Spectrum* took a team effort to write and publish. I would like to acknowledge those who encouraged and empowered me to write. My literary agent, Bob Hostetler, and the Steve Laube Agency team. Dr. Laurence A. Becker for sharing my journey with autism in his documentary film *Fierce Love and Art*. Miranda Keskes for editing my whole manuscript.

A special thanks to the individuals with autism who shared their stories in these pages: Tyler Gianchetta, Peter Lantz, Rachel Barcellona, Kimberly Dixon, Erik Weber, Chase Sibary, Becky Sharrock, Grandy Miller, Amanda LaMunyon, Walker Aurand, Haley Moss, Grant Manier, Seth Chwast, Malcolm Wang, Connor Keskes, William J. DeYonker, Alix Generous, Brittany Tagliareni, Tarik El-Abour, and Armani Williams.

Thanks to every parent and professional in the autism community whom I interviewed while writing this book: Barbara Barcellona, Jason Hague, Jim and Marilyn Dixon, Sandy Weber, Brian and Bina Sibary, Julie Coy, Brittany Miller, Sherry LaMunyon, Steve and Anne Walker, Karen Wang, Cathy Tagliareni, Nadia Khalil, and the countless others who helped.

I would like to thank my students at Destiny School of Ministry, and my coworkers at Havenwyck Hospital.

My thanks to the staff at Kregel Publications for their continual encouragement and desire to advance the gospel of Christ: Jerry Kregel,

Janyre Tromp, Sarah De Mey, Joel Armstrong, Catherine DeVries, Steve Barclift, Katherine Chappell, Phil Anderson, and Lori Alberda.

Finally, I would like to thank Jesus Christ for giving me the strength and grace to finish this project.

Extended Biographies of Select Featured Individuals

Rachel Barcellona is an autism advocate, model, author, singer, actress, and pageant winner. She is passionate about advocating for autism and encouraging those with disabilities to accomplish anything. "I show people that I can do anything despite my disability. Be yourself no matter what, and don't let others define who you are."
rachelbarcellona.com

William J. DeYonker began playing pool at the young age of four, but then converted to learning trick shots when he was fourteen. He is a top-ranked ESPN player and is currently ranked number one in the world! He travels around the United States and competes in nearly all trick shot competitions. Whenever he doesn't compete, he practices competitors' trick shots and spends most of his time creating new trick shots to take his artistry to the next level. The trick shots he creates are jaw-dropping and he is capable of performing over one thousand different shots!
willdeyonker.com

Kimberly Ruth Dixon was a published poet from Round Rock, Texas. Kimberly had nonverbal autism and communicated by typing. She enjoyed painting, riding horses, gardening, and starting conversations about great topics like dreams and religion. She also collected figurines:

dolls, birdhouses, jewelry, and crosses. She wrote a book of poetry and art: *Under the Silence Is Me—How It Feels to Be Nonverbal.* The book can be purchased at her Etsy store called kimsgifts.etsy.com. To learn more about this amazing woman's life, please visit the following sites.
freepoet85.weebly.com
facebook.com/KimberlyDixonAuthor

Amanda Grace LaMunyon is an artist from Enid, Oklahoma, diagnosed with Asperger's, who has savant abilities in painting and drawing. She sells her artwork, donating a portion of the sales to raise money for improving the lives of children with autism. Amanda's art has been displayed in galleries like the Salmagundi Club and Carnegie Hall in New York City and was featured on *The Today Show* with Megyn Kelly. She has received a number of state and national awards for community service in fundraising efforts for autism research and children's health.
amandalamunyon.com

Becky Sharrock enjoys speaking on the topics of human memory abilities, autism, and anxiety. She, with the help of her family, created a Facebook page for teens and adults with autism, where people with ASD can interact and feel supported. Becky also blogs about her experiences on her website, *A Life Journal: Dealing with Autism One Piece at a Time.*
alifejournaltalks.com
facebook.com/mylifeisapuzzle

Brittany Tagliareni was diagnosed with autism at an early age and regularly received a variety of therapies including occupational, speech, and physical. She began playing tennis at the age of sixteen and was drawn to the sport as a result of watching her brother, AJ, compete.

Brittany has the competitive heart of a champion and the desire that burns within all world-class athletes to achieve their goals. These character traits serve her well as she refuses to allow her autism and its physical, mental, and communicative manifestations to keep her from pursuing her dream of becoming a world champion tennis player.
brittanytagliareni.com

Malcolm Wang is an artist in Michigan. Malcolm was diagnosed with autism at age three. His artwork is sold through Mod Market in Northville, Michigan.

Erik N. Weber is a motivational speaker, author, and special education attorney. He represents students with special needs and their parents. He attends IEP meetings, reviews documents, conducts legal research, and informs parents of substantive and procedural rights in special education. Often, Erik performs these services pro bono. He is an appointed member of both the California Office of Administrative Hearings Special Education Advisory Committee and the California State Council on Developmental Disabilities.

Armani Williams is an eighteen-year-old Detroit-based professional NASCAR driver. Armani is part of the NASCAR stable of talented upcoming drivers. He is using his racing as a platform to draw more awareness to autism and create better life outcomes for families impacted by ASD. He competes for Calabrese Motor Sports and Flyin' Dutchman Racing.
teamarmaniracing.com

Notes

Introduction

1. Holly Robinson Peete, Ryan Elizabeth, and RJ Peete, *Same but Different: Teen Life on the Autism Express* (New York: Scholastic, 2018), 56.

2. Sarah Parshall Perry, *Sand in My Sandwich: And Other Motherhood Messes I'm Learning to Love* (Grand Rapids: Revell, 2015), 123.

3. Daniel R. Thomson, "A Biblical Disability-Ministry Perspective," in *Why, O God? Suffering and Disability in the Bible and Church*, ed. Larry J. Waters and Roy B. Zuck (Wheaton, IL: Crossway, 2011), 31.

4. Deborah Reber, *Differently Wired: Raising an Exceptional Child in a Conventional World* (New York: Workman, 2018), 57.

5. Stephanie O. Hubach, *Same Lake, Different Boat: Coming Alongside People Touched by Disability* (Phillipsburg, NJ: P&R, 2006), 29.

6. Ron Sandison, *A Parent's Guide to Autism: Practical Advice. Biblical Wisdom* (Lake Mary, FL: Charisma Media, 2016), 185. Additional information provided in an interview with Edie S. Brannigan on September 8, 2014. Used with permission.

7. "Mikey Brannigan: First Austistic American Runner to Win Paralympic 1500 Meter Gold, NBC Nightly News," NBC News, September 13, 2016, video, 2:05, https://youtu.be/keVZa_XmEcQ.

8. Peter A. Giersch, *Day by Day with St. Francis* (Totowa, NJ: Catholic Book Publishing, 2016), 82.

9. Diane Dokko Kim, *Unbroken Faith: Spiritual Recovery for the Special Needs Parent* (Franklin, TN: Worthy Publishing, 2017), 98.

10. Arthur Fleischmann with Carly Fleischmann, *Carly's Voice: Breaking Through Autism* (New York: Simon & Schuster, 2012), 193.
11. Augustine of Hippo, *Confessions*, trans. Maria Boulding (Hyde Park, NY: New City Press, 2007), 153.

Chapter 1: Real Superheroes Don't Wear Capes

1. Ann and Curt Warner with Dave Boling, *The Warner Boys: Our Family's Story of Autism and Hope* (New York: Little A, 2018), 88.
2. Fred R. Volkmar and Lisa A. Wiesner, *A Practical Guide to Autism: What Every Parent, Family Member, and Teacher Needs to Know* (Hoboken, NJ: John Wiley & Sons, 2009), 253.
3. "Autism Prevalence Rises in Communities Monitored by CDC," Centers for Disease Control and Prevention, April 16, 2020, https://www.cdc.gov /media/releases/2020/p0326-autism-prevalence-rises.html.
4. Temple Grandin, *The Way I See It: A Personal Look at Autism and Asperger's* (Arlington, TX: Future Horizons, 2008), 123.
5. I interviewed Tyler Gianchetta on October 14, 2015, and April 18, 2019. Used with permission.
6. Carolyn Gusoff, "Autistic Son Saves Mother from Burning Car on Long Island," CBS News, July 16, 2015, https://newyork.cbslocal.com/2015/07 /16/autistic-son-saves-mom-burning-car-li/.
7. Julie Hornok, "Three Steps to Finding Gratitude in the Trenches of Autism," *National Autism Association* (blog), November 20, 2018, https:// nationalautismassociation.org/three-steps-to-finding-gratitude-in-the -trenches-of-autism/. Used with permission.
8. Lori Ashley Taylor, *Dragonfly: A Daughter's Emergence from Autism* (New York: Skyhorse, 2018), 59.

Chapter 2: Where Hope Can Be Found

1. Austin John Jones, "Unsteadiness and Insecurity on the Autism Spectrum," The Art of Autism, May 31, 2018, https://the-art-of-autism.com/unsteadiness -and-insecurity-on-the-autism-spectrum/. Used with permission.
2. I interviewed Peter Lantz on June 20, 2018. Used with permission.
3. Stephane Kasriel, "The Future of Work Won't Be About College Degrees, It Will Be About Job Skills," CNBC, October 31, 2018, https://www.cnbc

.com/2018/10/31/the-future-of-work-wont-be-about-degrees-it-will-be
-about-skills.html.

4. Eric Metaxas, *Martin Luther: The Man Who Rediscovered God and Changed the World* (New York: Penguin, 2018), 316.

Chapter 3: Prairie Dogs and Honey Badgers

1. Pamela J. Wolfberg, *Play and Imagination in Children with Autism* (New York: Teachers College Press, 1999), 8.

2. Katherine Reynolds Lewis, *The Good News About Bad Behavior* (New York: Public Affairs, 2018), 12.

3. Whitney Ellenby, *Autism Uncensored* (Virginia Beach: Koehler Books, 2017), 212.

4. I interviewed Julie Hornok on December 3, 2018. Used with permission.

Chapter 4: Therapy Adventures

1. Moheb Costandi, *Neuroplasticity*, MIT Press Essential Knowledge Series (Cambridge, MA: MIT Press, 2016), 145–46.

2. Jessica Schrader, "Top Teacher Chelsea Campbell Reaches Kids with Kindness," *Metro Parent*, April 26, 2017, https://www.metroparent.com/m -school-issues/top-teacher-chelsea-campbell-reaches-kids-kindness/. Used with permission.

3. I interviewed Stephanie Holmes on October 3, 2016. Used with permission.

4. Rachel Summers, "Tips to Teach Autistic Children," The Art of Autism, January 11, 2018, https://the-art-of-autism.com/tips-to-teach-autistic -children/. Used with permission.

5. Sonu Khosla, "Important Strategies That Can Help Autistic Kids in the Classroom," *Autism Parenting Magazine*, June 24, 2020, https://www .autismparentingmagazine.com/strategies-helping-autistic-kids-in -classroom/.

6. Ron Sandison, "Autistic Man Creates Training Program That Allows Others with Autism to Overcome Anxiety, Depression, and Social Limitations," The Art of Autism, June 27, 2017, https://the-art-of-autism.com /autistic-man-creates-training-program-that-allows-others-with-autism -to-overcome-anxiety-depression-and-social-limitations/.

7. I interviewed Jeremy Samson on January 27, 2017. Used with permission.

8. I interviewed Anthony Ianni on June 27, 2018. Used with permission.

9. Lisa Jo Rudy, *Get Out, Explore, and Have Fun!* (Philadelphia: Jessica Kingsley Publishers, 2010), 21, 24.

10. I interviewed Brittany Miller on May 28, 2019. Used with permission.

Chapter 5: Gifts to Be Found

1. Judith Newman, *To Siri with Love: A Mother, Her Autistic Son, and the Kindness of Machines* (New York: HarperCollins, 2017), 206.

2. "Titanic Exclusive Display," Pigeon Forge Tennessee, accessed February 24, 2021, https://www.mypigeonforge.com/event/titanic-lego-display.

3. Caitlin O'Kane, "Autistic Boy Overcomes Obstacles to Build Largest Lego Replica of the Titanic," CBS News, April 25, 2018, https://www.cbsnews .com/news/autistic-boy-overcomes-obstacles-to-build-largest-lego -replica-of-the-titanic/.

4. Ron Sandison, "William J. DeYonker: Three-Time Billiard Trick Shot Champion," The Art of Autism, September 23, 2019, https://the-art-of -autism.com/william-j-deyonker-three-time-billiard-trick-shot-master -champion/. Used with permission.

Chapter 6: Painted Butterfly

1. Elizabeth M. Bonker and Virginia G. Breen, *I Am in Here* (Grand Rapids: Revell, 2011), 70.

2. Kathie Maximovich, "Breaking boundaries is one of the ways we experience life to its fullest potential," Facebook, August 17, 2020. Used with permission.

3. J. Lamar Hardwick, "How Our 'Thorns' Make Us Better," *The Autism Pastor* (blog), November 25, 2018, http://autismpastor.com/?p=2738.

4. N. T. Wright, *Surprised by Hope: Rethinking Heaven, the Resurrection, and the Mission of the Church* (New York: HarperOne, 2018), 213.

5. Augustine of Hippo, *Confessions*, trans. Maria Boulding (Hyde Park, NY: New City Press, 2007), 122.

6. I interviewed Marilyn and Jim Dixon, Kimberly Dixon's parents, on August 1, 2017, and December 3, 2018. Used with permission. Kimberly Dixon's poems and writing were provided to the author by Marilyn and Jim Dixon. All materials used with permission.

7. Thomas à Kempis, *The Imitation of Christ* (London: Penguin, 1987), 83.

8. Kimberly Dixon's moving story is featured in Dr. Laurence A. Becker's 2017 documentary film *Fierce Love and Art*.

Chapter 7: Fierce Love and Art

1. Ron Sandison, "Fierce Love and Art: An Interview with Dr. Laurence Becker," The Art of Autism, July 3, 2017, https://the-art-of-autism.com/fierce-love-and-art-an-interview-with-dr-laurence-becker/.

2. Mariale Hardiman, Susan Magsamen, Guy McKhann, and Janet Eilber, "Neuroeducation: Learning, Arts, and the Brain: Findings and Challenges for Educators and Researchers from the 2009 Johns Hopkins University Summit," Americans for the Arts, 2009, 58, https://www.americansforthearts.org/by-program/reports-and-data/legislation-policy/naappd/neuroeducation-learning-arts-and-the-brain.

3. Claire Draycot, "Using Art and Creativity to Engage an Autistic Child in the Classroom," The Art of Autism, June 16, 2018, https://the-art-of-autism.com/educating-autism-art-and-creativity-to-engage-an-autistic-child-in-the-classroom/. Used with permission.

4. Lisa Jo Rudy, "How Art Therapy Helps People with Autism," Verywell Health, April 28, 2019, https://www.verywellhealth.com/art-therapy-for-autism-260054.

5. Mark Lewis Wagner, "Ten Reasons Art Is Good for Kids and the World," Drawing on the Earth, 2015, https://drawingonearth.org/resources/10-reasons-why/.

6. Wagner, "Ten Reasons Art Is Good."

7. I interviewed Haley Moss on June 12, 2019. Used with permission.

8. Debra Chwast, *An Unexpected Life: A Mother and Son's Story of Love, Determination, Autism, and Art* (New York: Sterling, 2011), 13.

9. Chwast, *An Unexpected Life*, 128.

10. Mary Bowerman, "Was a Saudi Prince the Mystery Buyer of $450 Million Leonardo Da Vinci Painting?" *USA Today*, December 7, 2017, https://www.usatoday.com/story/news/nation-now/2017/12/07/saudi-prince-mystery-buyer-450-million-leonardo-da-vinci-painting/929856001/.

11. "Modern Living: Ozmosis in Central Park," *Time*, October 4, 1976, http://content.time.com/time/subscriber/article/0,33009,918412,00.html.

12. George Viereck, "What Life Means to Einstein," *Saturday Evening Post*, October 26, 1929, https://www.saturdayeveningpost.com/wp-content /uploads/satevepost/what_life_means_to_einstein.pdf.

13. G. K. Chesterton, *The Everlasting Man* (Peabody, MA: Hendrickson, 2007), 100. First published 1925.

Chapter 8: Excellent Choices

1. I interviewed Diane Dokko Kim on April 23, 2018. Used with permission.

2. Karla Akins, *A Pair of Miracles: A Story of Autism, Faith, and Determined Parenting* (Grand Rapids: Kregel, 2017), 37.

3. I interviewed Terry Pagliei on May 31, 2019. Used with permission.

4. Ethan Hirschberg, "How Parents Can Help Their Children on the Spectrum," *The Journey Through Autism* (blog), May 12, 2019, https://www .thejourneythroughautism.com/single-post/2019/05/12/How-Parents-Can -Help-Their-Children-On-The-Spectrum. Used with permission.

5. Used with permission from Miranda Keskes. And a huge thank you to Miranda, who did the initial edit of this book.

6. I interviewed Rachel Barcellona on June 29, 2015, and May 16, 2019. Used with permission.

Chapter 9: Fear Not

1. Laura Kasbar's story appears in Julie Hornok, *United in Autism: Finding Strength Inside the Spectrum* (Dallas: Brown Books, 2018), 94, 96.

2. Henri Nouwen, *Here and Now* (New York: Crossroad, 1994), 33.

3. Anne Moore Burnett, *Step Ahead of Autism: What You Can Do to Ensure the Best Possible Outcome for Your Child* (Forest Lake, MN: Sunrise River, 2011), 93.

4. Maritza A. Molis, *Autism in Our Home: The Making of a Bittersweet Family* (Meadville, PA: Christian Faith Publishing, 2018), 51.

5. Amy Mason, "The Key to Living a Courageous Life," *Amy Mason's Blog* (blog), January 31, 2018, http://www.amyemason.com/blog-1/2018/1/31 /the-key-to-living-a-courageous-life.

6. Janet Lintala with Martha W. Murphy, *The Un-Prescription for Autism: A Natural Approach for a Calmer, Happier, and More Focused Child* (New York: Amacom, 2016), 75–76.

7. I interviewed Amanda Grace LaMunyon on October 6, 2018. Used with permission.

8. This version of the poem was emailed from Amanda Grace LaMunyon to me on October 27, 2018. Used with permission.

Chapter 10: That's Life

1. Myroslaw Tataryn and Maria Truchan-Tataryn, *Discovering Trinity in Disability: A Theology for Embracing Difference* (Maryknoll, NY: Orbis, 2013), 50.

2. Thomas E. Reynolds, *Vulnerable Communion: A Theology of Disabilities and Hospitality* (Grand Rapids: Brazos, 2008), 51–52.

3. Deborah Reber, *Differently Wired: Raising an Exceptional Child in a Conventional World* (New York: Workman Publishing, 2018), 45.

4. Marina Sarris, "Stress and the Autism Parent," Interactive Autism Network, April 6, 2017, https://iancommunity.org/ssc/stress-and-autism-parent.

5. Angela Gachassin, *Autism: Healed for Life* (Bloomington, IN: WestBow, 2018), 17.

6. Charles Haddon Spurgeon, *The Salt-Cellars: Being a Collection of Proverbs, Together with Homely Notes Thereon*, vol. 1 (London: Passmore and Alabaster, 1889), 89.

7. Andrew and Rachel Wilson, *The Life We Never Expected* (Wheaton, IL: Crossway, 2016), 64.

8. Mother Teresa, *A Simple Path* (New York: Ballantine, 1995), 7.

9. C. T. Lewis, *The Sanctuary of the Soul* (Bloomington, IN: WestBow, 2013), 122.

10. Julie Hornok, *United in Autism: Finding Strength Inside the Spectrum* (Dallas: Brown Books, 2018), 120.

11. Stephen J. Bedard, *How to Make Your Church Autism-Friendly* (self-pub., CreateSpace, 2016), 24.

12. Rachel Marie Martin, *The Brave Art of Motherhood: Fight Fear, Gain Confidence, and Find Yourself Again* (Colorado Springs: WaterBrook, 2018), 145.

Chapter 11: Learning to Communicate

1. Anita Lesko, *Becoming an Autism Success Story* (Arlington, TX: Future Horizons, 2019), 103–5.

2. Temple Grandin, *The Way I See It: A Personal Look at Autism and Asperger's* (Arlington, TX: Future Horizons, 2008), 225.

3. Arthur Fleischmann with Carly Fleischmann, *Carly's Voice: Breaking Through Autism* (New York: Simon & Schuster, 2012), 233–34.

4. Katherine Reynolds Lewis, *The Good News About Bad Behavior* (New York: Public Affairs, 2018), 25.

5. I interviewed Brian and Bina Sibary on July 29, 2019. Used with permission.

Chapter 12: Capturing the Moment

1. Margot Sunderland, "The Science Behind How Holidays Make Your Child Happier—and Smarter," *Telegraph*, February 1, 2017, https://www.telegraph.co.uk/travel/family-holidays/the-science-behind-how-holidays-make-your-child-happier-and-smarter/.

2. Anne K. Fishel, *Home for Dinner: Mixing Food, Fun, and Conversation for a Happier Family and Healthier Kids* (New York: Amacom, 2015), 7.

3. I interviewed Jason Hague on December 22, 2018. Used with permission.

4. I interviewed Malcolm Wang and Karen Wang on March 16, 2018, and January 5, 2019. Used with permission.

Chapter 13: Living the Dream

1. Marc Gellman, "An Argument Against Happiness," *Newsweek*, October 4, 2006, https://www.newsweek.com/gellman-argument-against-happiness-111475.

2. Steve Greene, *Love Leads: The Spiritual Connection Between Your Relationships and Productivity* (Lake Mary, FL: Charisma House, 2017), 211.

3. "Harvard Psychologists Reveal Parents Who Raise Good Kids Do These 6 Things," *Health Food House*, December 21, 2018, https://www.healthyfoodhouse.com/harvard-psychologists-reveal-parents-who-raise-good-kids-do-these-6-things/.

4. Stella Acquarone, quoted in Jessica Hewitson, *Autism: How to Raise a Happy Autistic Child* (London: Orion Spring, 2018), 123.

5. Kaitlyn Alanis, "Bullied Boy with Different-Colored Eyes, Cleft Lip Rescues Cat with Same Rare Condition," *Wichita Eagle*, April 1, 2018, https://www.kansas.com/news/nation-world/national/article207615999

.html. (It's worth your time to look up pictures of this beautiful boy and his kitty.)

6. Anita Lesko, *Becoming an Autism Success Story* (Arlington, TX: Future Horizons, 2019), 53.

7. "Human-Animal Bond," American Veterinary Medical Association, accessed February 24, 2021, https://www.avma.org/one-health/human -animal-bond.

8. Robert Holden, *Be Happy: Release the Power of Happiness in You* (Carlsbad, CA: Hay House, 2009).

9. I interviewed Alix Generous on December 3, 2015, and January 26, 2019. Used with permission.

10. Raymond B. Fosdick, *Cumberland Alumnus* 9, no. 1 (September 1929): 3.

11. Alix Generous, "How I Learned to Communicate My Inner Life with Asperger's," TEDWomen, June 2015, video, 10:11, https://www.ted.com /talks/alix_generous_how_i_learned_to_communicate_my_inner_life _with_asperger_s?language=en.

Chapter 14: First Gleam of Dawn

1. Ron Sandison, *A Parent's Guide to Autism: Practical Advice. Biblical Wisdom* (Lake Mary, FL: Charisma Media, 2016), 184. Additional information provided in an interview with Edie S. Brannigan on September 8, 2014. Used with permission.

2. Maria Hechanova, "Avondale Autistic Barber Inspires Others to Overcome Their Fears," *Arizona's Family News*, May 23, 2019, https://www.azfamily .com/news/features/avondale-autistic-barber-inspires-others-to-overcome -their-fears/article_250e559a-7d7e-11e9-8376-eb72acef009c.html.

3. I interviewed Cathy Tagliareni and Brittany Tagliareni on June 7, 2019. I first published this article as "Meet Brittany Tagliareni, Slayer of Giants on the Tennis Court," The Art of Autism, August 11, 2019, https://the-art -of-autism.com/meet-brittany-tagliareni-slayer-of-giants-on-the-tennis -court/. Used with permission.

Chapter 15: Empowerment for Parenting Endurance

1. I interviewed Walker Aurand on December 17, 2018. Used with permission.

2. Martin Kessler, "For Walker Aurand, Hockey Was the Right Therapy for Autism," WBUR.org, May 8, 2020, https://www.wbur.org/onlyagame /2016/11/04/walker-aurand-davenport-university-hockey.

Chapter 16: Soaring as Eagles

1. I interviewed Julie Hornok on December 3, 2018. Used with permission.
2. I interviewed Erik N. Weber and Sandy Weber on December 13, 2018. Used with permission.

Chapter 17: God's Got This

1. Steve Jobs, "'You've Got to Find What You Love,' Jobs Says," Stanford News, June 14, 2005, https://news.stanford.edu/2005/06/14/jobs -061505/.
2. Philip Yancey, *Prayer: Does It Make Any Difference?* (Grand Rapids: Zondervan, 2016), 210.
3. Scripture taken from *The Message.* Copyright © 1993, 1994, 1995, 1996, 2000, 2001, 2002 by Eugene H. Peterson. Used by permission of NavPress. All rights reserved. Represented by Tyndale House Publishers, Inc.
4. Jason Hague, *Aching Joy: Following God Through the Land of Unanswered Prayer* (Colorado Springs: NavPress, 2018), 195.
5. O. Ivar Lovaas, *Teaching Developmentally Disabled Children: The Me Book* (Austin: PRO-ED, 1981), 165.
6. Oswald Chambers, "Something More About His Ways," My Utmost for His Highest, accessed February 24, 2021, https://utmost.org/classic /something-more-about-his-ways-classic/.
7. "Wave Hello to the Surf Genius with Asperger's," *Independent*, October 3, 2009, https://www.independent.co.uk/life-style/health-and-families /features/wave-hello-to-the-surf-genius-with-aspergers-1797025.html.

Chapter 18: Eternal Perspective

1. I interviewed Becky Sharrock on July 11, 2018. Used with permission.

Chapter 19: Answers to Prayers

1. Søren Kierkegaard, *Provocations: Spiritual Writings of Kierkegaard* (Walden, NY: Plough Publishing, 2014), 311.

2. Jason Hague, *Aching Joy: Following God Through the Land of Unanswered Prayer* (Colorado Springs: NavPress, 2018), 178.

3. Oswald Chambers, "The Purpose of Prayer," My Utmost for His Highest, accessed February 24, 2021, https://utmost.org/the-purpose-of-prayer/.

4. Augustine of Hippo, *Confessions*, trans. Maria Boulding (Hyde Park, NY: New City Press, 2007), 234.

5. Steve and Miranda Keskes shared the story of their son Connor with me on August 8, 2020. Used with permission.

Chapter 20: Ain't No Stoppin' Us Now

1. Patrick Marlborough, "Depression Steals Your Soul and Then It Takes Your Friends," Vice, January 31, 2017, https://www.vice.com/en/article /4x4xjj/depression-steals-your-soul-and-then-it-takes-your-friends. Used with permission.

2. "How Great Is Our God" is a CCM worship song from Chris Tomlin's 2004 album *Arriving*. "Awesome God" is a worship song from Richard Mullins's 1988 album *Winds of Heaven, Stuff of Earth*.

3. I interviewed Nadia Khalil on February 7, 2019. Used with permission.

4. Jeffrey Flanagan, "Royals Sign El-Abour, Outfielder with Autism," MLB .com, April 13, 2018, https://www.mlb.com/royals/news/tarik-el-abour -autistic-outfielder-signs-c272058962.

Chapter 21: The Race Marked Out for Us

1. Deborah Reber, *Differently Wired: Raising an Exceptional Child in a Conventional World* (New York: Workman, 2018), 246.

2. I interviewed Julie Hornok on December 3, 2018. Used with permission.

3. Christopher Bergland, "3 Specific Ways That Helping Others Benefits Your Brain," Psychology Today, February 21, 2016, https://www.psychol ogytoday.com/us/blog/the-athletes-way/201602/3-specific-ways-helping -others-benefits-your-brain.

4. Devon Still with Mark Dagostino, *Still in the Game: Finding the Faith to Tackle Life's Biggest Challenges* (Nashville: Thomas Nelson, 2018), 197.

5. I interviewed Armani Williams on August 27, 2018. Used with permission.

6. Davey Segal, "Armani Williams Defying the Odds and Living His Dream in NASCAR," Hometracks, August 20, 2018, https://hometracks.nascar

.com/2018/08/20/armani-williams-defying-the-odds-and-living-his -dream-in-nascar/. Used with permission.

Conclusion

1. "Autism Advocate Dani Bowman at Temple Grandin & Friends," Goody-Awards, May 21, 2015, video, 4:52, https://youtu.be/Tsfq1KMIkU8.

2. Judith Newman, *To Siri with Love: A Mother, Her Autistic Son, and the Kindness of Machines* (New York: HarperCollins, 2017), xvii.

3. Haley Moss's keynote presentation at Milestones Autism Conference, Cleveland, Ohio, on June 12, 2019. Used with permission.

For weary parents of kids with special
needs from a parent who's been there

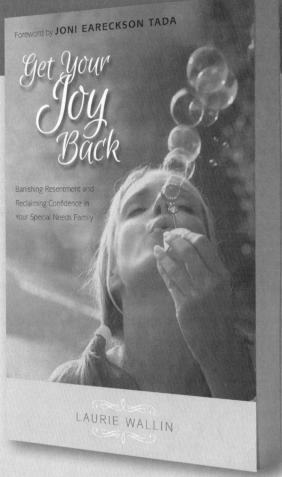

"*Get Your Joy Back* is unique in that it is written to teach
parents how to care for themselves *so that they can truly care
for their children*. . . . Wallin sugarcoats nothing but addresses
issues with honesty, humor, and—above all—hope."
—*Christian Living*

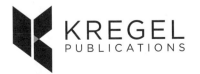

"Kelly Langston takes our hand and walks us through the giant of autism with the strength and conviction of David when he slew Goliath."
—*Libraries Alive*

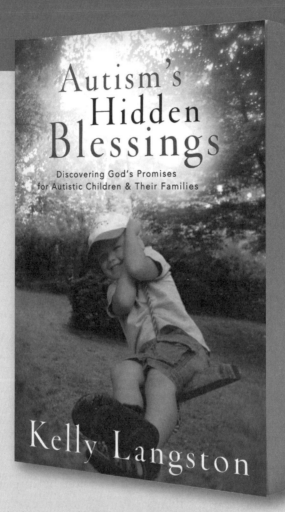

Through the story of her own ongoing struggles and victories raising her autistic son, Kelly Langston brings to light God's promises for exceptional kids and assures parents of their children's potential and beauty.

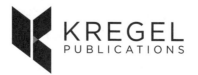

KREGEL
PUBLICATIONS